THE TEENAGER'S GUIDE TO UNDERSTANDING & MANAGING WEIGHT:

Questions, Answers, Tips, & Cautions

Michael D. LeBow, Ph.D., C. Psych.

Science & Humanities Press

Chesterfield Missouri USA

Publication Date, March, 2012

ISBN 9781596300729

Library of Congress Control Number: 2011939296

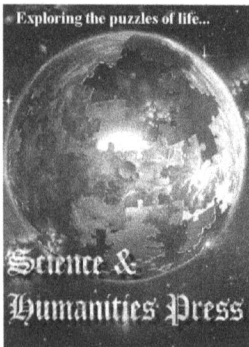

Science & Humanities Press

PO Box 7151

Chesterfield, MO 63006-7151

sciencehumanitiespress.com

Dedication:

To George Miskovsky and Bill Potts

Your kindness and determination turned my loss of over 50 years, into my treasure of today.

Other Books on Weight, Overweight, & Obesity by Michael LeBow:

If only I were thin (with R. Perry)

Weight control: The behavioral strategies

Child obesity: A new frontier of behavior therapy

The thin plan

Adult obesity therapy

Overweight children

Overweight teenagers: Don't bear the burden alone

Dieter's Snake Pit

Acknowledgments

I wish I could thank each erudite behavioral scientist who has over the years influenced my thinking and, as result, this book. Two, Drs. David Burns and Aaron Beck, in particular have showed me and other clinicians that what people tell themselves profoundly affects their feelings and behavior. Think better to feel better.

I wish also to acknowledge the impact that the CDC centers for disease control and the choosemyplate website have had on the writing of this book.

Finally, I wish to acknowledge Dr. Bud Banis, head of Science and Humanities Press, for his continual support and encouragement. Without his backing and timely commentary, this work would never have reached fruition.

Contents

INTRODUCTION

It was freezing that Tuesday afternoon. But what really chilled me to my bones was 15-year-old Callie Corcoran's icy declaration. Sitting across from me, eyes fixed on mine, determined, she said, "I'd rather be dead than fat again." I knew she meant it.

From grade 4 to grade 9, she had struggled with weight and now had resolved to no longer struggle again, no matter what. Her words scared me—so drastic, so final, so horrible, so unnecessary. Sadly though, they do echo those of many other teenagers, some heavy and some not.

Fortunately, after having talked through her issues, Callie now thinks better of herself and more realistically about her weight, whatever it may become. No longer does she claim, as do some of her peers, magazines, and TV programs, that you are what you weigh—nothing else, nothing more. But you are more, far more. Callie would tell you to untie your feelings of self-worth from pounds on a scale, if you don't believe you're more. She'd also tell you that if you are overweight or obese do something about it, just make sure what you do is smart and healthy.

This book shows you exactly what smart and healthy mean. **First**, it answers questions about weight, overweight, and obesity. You learn:

- how to find out if you really are too heavy, and what too heavy means

- what teenagers face if they are too heavy

- why, possibly, some teenagers can eat anything and everything and yet not gain extra weight

- where online to find the best advice about what and how much to eat

- what calories truly are

- what the difference is between energy and energetic

- why to become more active

- why a teenager becomes too heavy

- when heavy teenagers should not lose weight, and what to do instead

- what the body mass index (BMI) is & how to measure yours

- what drives weight bullying

- and much much more

Second, the book offers practical and health-preserving tips on how to manage weight well—52 of them. These carefully explained guides range from eating smarter and moving more to thinking upbeat thoughts about yourself and talking back to weight bullies. Here's just a sample of the 52 tips:

- #1 Shine a Light on Your Eating.

- #2 Explore Choosemyplate.

- #11 Trick Some of Your Snack Attacks.

- #16 Make Snacks Chewier by Adding Vegetables or Fruit To Them So They Last Longer.

- #26 Retrain Your Brain: Take Smaller Portions *at Home & Restaurants.*

- #27 Retrain Your Brain: Take Fewer Helpings.

- #28 Retrain Your Brain: Eat When Hungry, Stop When Full.

2

- #29 Let Moderate Hunger Guide You.

- #34 Move More Each Day, Every day—at least 60 minutes more.

- #36 Make A Weekly Activity Plan.

- #37 Get Paid for Progress.

- # 41 Talk back to Those Who Bring You Down: Others & Yourself..

Third, the book lists 20 cautions. Understanding and heeding most if not all of them is a must. To help you manage your weight sensibly, healthfully, and safely, some cautions focus on what to do *before* starting a weight management program, such as talking to a doctor. Others zero-in on what to do *after* beginning the program, such as sidestepping snakes of weight mismanagement.

Fourth, the book offers a message the following true story illustrates:

It was 1943. WWII was still raging and taking young American lives.

My father, then in his mid-30s with two children and a pregnant wife, was drafted into the Navy; he would serve the next 18 months as a Navy corpsman. Before he boarded the train to his faraway destination, my mother gave him a stylish solid silver identification bracelet. It had a thick 2 inch long silver nameplate that attached on its right and left to large heavy interlocking links; a silver clasp locked the bracelet around his wrist. Engraved on the front was his name "Bill LeBow," and on the back my mothers first name "Mildred"; actually, she had "Love Mildred" engraved. For my father, the bracelet was a reminder of my mother's love.

When he did eventually return, he regaled my mother with stories of beautiful Southern California, convincing her that therein lay the promised land for us. It wasn't hard to sell that idea to her, because she hated the winters in Detroit, the city where we lived then, and would have no qualms about watching the place gradually disappear from view as we drove the 3000 miles west to our new home. That trip for me at the age of four was punishing. I was cramped for four long days in the backseat of our uncomfortably warm car sitting beside my eight-year-old sister Esty; the two of us battled each other continually. The car smelled of soured milk, and we all were regularly jostled up and down on the many bumpy roads and frightened on the treacherously narrow winding mountainous paths; I was carsick throughout the ordeal. But eventually we arrived in California.

To my mother, life was easier there than it had been in Detroit. One way it was, she realized a few months after arriving, was no longer having to layer her children with binding cold-climate apparel every winter. We could go outside without it and return home without having to remove it. And we could do this repeatedly throughout the day. California winters were hardly noticeable. Detroit winters, on the other hand, were literally in-your-face, inescapable, harsh, and often cruel.

Unaware of how much I had always admired my father's identification bracelet, my mother showed it to me one day in 1954 while reorganizing her jewelry box. It was being stored there, she said, for safekeeping. "I gave this to Dad in 1943 just after he was drafted; I knew the story well but enjoyed hearing it retold. Couldn't have him forgetting me now, could I," she

4

said, and then smiled. She knew I knew that the likelihood of his forgetting her was 100 times less than the chance of his finding $1 million worth of diamonds buried in our backyard while mowing the lawn. To him, the bracelet had been and still was A SOLID SILVER SYMBOL of their love.

After she said this, when I saw it in the box, my admiration of it mushroomed into desire for it. I had to have it. It had always looked good on my father's wrist and I just knew it would look good on mine, too. I wanted it, but clearly had no right to it. Yet, my intense desire for it allowed me to easily put that moral concern aside. To my 12 year old, soon to be 13-year-old eyes, the bracelet was manly, a sign of power. So, collecting my courage, I asked, more like begged, Dad for it. Considering my plea and discussing it with Mom, he, nice guy that he was, agreed to it and even let me have the bracelet re-engraved and resized to fit my wrist.

On the front, I put **Mike LeBow** and on the back linked my name with those of the special four I lived with at that time in my life, **Mom and Dad** and my sisters, **Julie** and **Esty**. Though he never said so, I knew that Dad wasn't just giving me the bracelet, he was entrusting me with it. I silently vowed never to let it leave my wrist. Forever would it remain there, I was certain. It was to me, after all, A SOLID SILVER SYMBOL of my dad's trust.

That summer in 1954, my uncle invited Julie, now 10 years old, and I to join him and his family for a week of camping at beautiful Lake Tahoe in Northern California. We flew on a propeller airplane—jet planes weren't as yet all that common— 400 miles to their San Francisco home. The next morning, we seven would-be campers piled into my uncle's Jaguar sedan for the

5

scenic half day trip to South Lake Tahoe. As we got closer to our destination, the landscape changed from homes, city streets, and shops to a forest of pine trees so tall your neck would hurt when you tried to see their tops and so refreshing your lungs never wanted to exhale their wonderful sent. Lake Tahoe is paradise. During our week there, we swam daily until our ears clogged up and our bellies churned with hunger. We cooked our meals on a Coleman stove, slept soundly and warmly all night inside zippered sleeping bags atop air mattresses carefully placed in a tent, awakened each morning to find water frozen in the buckets, breakfasted on hotcakes dripping with butter and maple syrup, and when the sun had sufficiently warmed the air—usually by noon— raced the hundred or so yards from our campsite to the lake to swim and dog-paddle about in its icy water. This was our routine all the time we were there.

Often I'd check to see that my most prized possession was still was where it was supposed to be— on my left wrist. Our last day of camping started out warmer than usual, so not to miss a minute of good weather, we arrived on the Tahoe shore earlier than usual. I enjoyed the lake for about an hour before needing to leave it and warm up. My bracelet, I'm almost positive, was on my wrist when I lay on my towel.

Within 10 minutes, almost asleep, I heard, "Michael, Michael, help me." It was Julie. Startled, though groggy, I jumped up and ran into the lake. As soon as the frigid water hit me, I was jolted further into consciousness, and swam speedily to my sister. It turned out that she wasn't in a lot of trouble, just tired and finding it difficult to swim. So I guided her back to shore as she held onto me. Moments after Julie and I left the water, my aunt declared that I had saved my sister, but I knew my aunt was exaggerating and probably just kidding. Nonetheless, her words made me feel good. That feeling, however, vanished in a heartbeat, for when I looked down, I saw only white skin on my left wrist. My bracelet was gone.

Two hundred volts of electricity coursed through me, burning me, grabbing me, holding on to me. My bracelet was gone.

Shock, frantic, queasy. I wanted to sob, but held back. Maybe it was on my blanket. Maybe I had dropped it in the sand. I silently prayed, *Please let me find it. Please God, let me find it.* Then I bargained: *I'll try harder at school. I'll bring home A's. I'll stop fighting with Esty (age 17). I'll be nice to her, even when she's a snake.*

My cousins, aunt and uncle, Julie, even a few fellow sunbathers, helped me search the sand. Nothing. I dived into the lake oblivious now to its cold and ran my fingers through its soggy floor everywhere I thought my feet had been, all the while hoping and hoping and hoping.

Still nothing. The bracelet was gone, my hopes of finding it demolished.

The dictionary defines "devastate" as to lay waste to, to ravage, to overpower, to overcome, to overwhelm. I felt worse than devastated. On the plane back to LA, my mind raced with, *What do I tell Dad? Will he think I'm a jerk, a screw-up? Will he ever again trust me?* Once home I tearfully recounted the gory details and waited for his anger, disappointment, and disgust. They didn't come. He frowned, but didn't explode, not even a "you dummy-look", or side to side headshake of "I knew it", or an exasperated "Oh Michael." Not even an annoyed "Oh, Michael." Throughout all his time in the Navy, throughout all he had faced, he had kept that bracelet safe. Afterwards for years at work selling numerous products, at home doing chores, at play tossing baseballs and footballs back and forth with me, he had kept that bracelet safe. He had worn it everywhere; it hadn't been stored in the jewelry box for very long. For 11 years, he had kept that bracelet safe. I couldn't do it for much longer than 11 days. Couldn't he at least let me have a grumpy *"Oh, Michael."*

He didn't. Sometimes *nice* hurts more than *nasty*. I felt really lousy and low. His concern was only for my well-being, only about how I felt having lost something I cared about so much. That was the man he was. I realized soon that it was me who was angry, disappointed, and disgusted, not my father. Three years later a massive heart attack took him away from me and any chance I may have had to redeem myself; even if he didn't need me to, I did.

Eventually I forgot the bracelet episode. There were new challenges to meet: my senior year of high school, college, and eventually graduate school. After earning my doctorate and marrying, I moved with my wife to Winnipeg where I became a practicing clinical psychologist and professor of psychology at the University of Manitoba.

Several years later I did something very important to this story without realizing it at the time. Not remembering the bracelet at all, I once again linked the special people in my life to me. This time I did that, not by engraving their names on valuable jewelry as I had done so many years ago, but by dedicating my first book to them—mom, dad, Julie, and Esty.

The book came out in 1973. It would be almost 35 years later before I learned how significant that dedication would prove to be.

Tuesday, August 14, 2007. As my body so often does, my power wheel chair was refusing to follow my commands. Its defiance had just caused me to skin my knuckles on the door jam to my office as I was trying to wheel my way in. Adding insult to injury, 25 pages of my notes lay strewn on my office floor. While trying to soothe my very red, very scraped and very sore knuckles, I clumsily had knocked the papers from my desk to the floor. Picking them up would take about 25 minutes, I don't bend so easily anymore and lately had little energy. Worst of all on that Tuesday in November, the feelings of hopelessness about being disabled, feelings I battle regularly and hate passionately, were once again chewing on me.

So no wonder that it wasn't until I reached with my mechanical pincher to retrieve a few of the pages from the floor directly beneath my phone that I noticed the phone's nagging *you've got voicemail* light blinking. "If you're Mike LeBow call Placerville California," said the disembodied voice in the message. " We have found valuable jewelry of yours in South Lake Tahoe. "

"Come on," I said to myself, "what an obvious scam, a dumb one, too. How many people in Winnipeg have been to Lake Tahoe, let alone lost jewelry there." I had not thought about the missing bracelet for years and not even the mention of Lake Tahoe and found jewelry could revive that old painful memory quite yet. My only thought at the moment was "I wonder what they'll try to sell me." Curious, I put common sense aside and returned the call. At least it wasn't a 900 number.

George Miskovsky answered on the third ring, and I said, "You called me about some jewelry you found. I'm Dr. Michael LeBow.

"Did you lose a silver bracelet a couple of years ago in Lake Tahoe?", he asked.

"No," "I haven't been there in over a half century." Now recalling bracelet incident I added, "I did lose a man's identification bracelet back then, but that was so long ago, it has probably disintegrated."

"Well," George responded, "you're Mike LeBow aren't you? Your name is on the front of it."

But there must be a lot of Mike LeBow's I said to myself, beginning to accept that maybe this was no scam.

"There' s writing on the back, too, 'Mom and Dad, Julie and Esty'."

Now I was certain this was no scam, but still wondered how in the world could he possibly have a bracelet that Lake Tahoe had swallowed 53 years ago?

Nonetheless, it felt as if a burden I had been carrying was beginning to lift. Within a week George's computer-savvy boss, Bill Potts, e-mailed a digital picture of the bracelet to me. There it was, front and back. That was really it, and the weight on me of having lost a valuable treasure my father had entrusted to me was fading.

From Bill, I learned that George's hobby is regularly sweeping parts of the lake with his mettle detector to uncover its buried treasures which he then returns to their rightful owners. Mine, he had unearthed from deep in the lake about 30 feet from shore. For months, he and Bill had been searching for

10

me in order to return the bracelet. Lots of Mike LeBows out there evidently. To narrow the search and therefore improve results, they eventually had added my sisters' names, Julie and Esty, engraved on the back of the bracelet. That clue had led them to the 1973 dedication of my first book to my sisters and subsequently, with a little more digging, to me. I wanted to pay George for finding the bracelet and cover the charges for returning it to me. "No", he said firmly. "No reward, and I'll send it to you."

Some people get great pleasure from being kind to others. They belong to a club that certainly could use a few more members. All that George wanted was for me to write down the history of the bracelet and how I felt having it again after all these years. So, I did. I wrote how it began as a solid silver symbol to my dad of the love he and my mother shared, and how it later became a solid silver symbol to me of my father's trust. I also wrote to George about my despair over having lost it, and my fear that by doing so I had let my father down and lost his trust. I also told him about feeling hopeless about ever finding the bracelet and how unburdening my seeing it again was to me.

Finally, I told George that the bracelet will always be my solid silver reminder that when my inabilities seem unmanageable and my disabilities insurmountable to never give up hope. That's the message this story has for me.

As I was writing the letter I thought also, but didn't say, that this is the sort of story my dad would have loved to hear, the sort of story that I know would have put a smile on his face. Maybe, I thought, just maybe my dad, lost to me for so many years, was smiling.

Four decades ago when I was learning to be a clinical psychologist, a wise professor told me that the most important thing therapists can give their patients is hope. He went on to say that having hope motivates those seeking help to work harder and longer at changing their lives for the better. My old professor was right. Never give up hope. That's a four word truth the bracelet story helps me remember and one I want you to never forget.

Be mindful of the four words, especially if you're a teenager who's overweight or obese and who feels helpless or hopeless about the chances of doing something about it. Many young people have altered their lifestyles to healthfully overcome their weight problems. Even if you have tried before but been unable to do that or even if you believe your condition is too long-standing and too complex to do that, never give up hope.

~~

The Teenager's Guide can help you. It's packed with information that will enable you to understand what you're up against. And it is packed with tools that will enable you to sensibly and healthfully take charge and stay in charge of your weight every day. This book will show you how to do this important job the right way.

12

Chapter 1:
Name-calling and Character-bashing

As you'll read and unfortunately may already know first hand, many heavy teens are blamed, shamed, and teased day in and day out for being heavy. They're accused of gluttony, laziness, and weakness for no reason other than looking heavy. Chapter 1 talks about this name-calling and character-bashing and suggests what to do about the weight bullies and weight blamers who champion it.

IF YOU'RE TOO HEAVY IS IT BECAUSE YOU EAT TOO MUCH?

Short answer: NOT NECESSARILY

Some heavy teenagers routinely down huge meals and humongous snacks, but not all heavy teenagers do. The same can be said for thin teenagers. Some regularly pack-in nachos, sweet rolls, onion rings, guacamole dip, french-fries, teen burgers, but not all do. So, clearly, the overeating explanation just doesn't apply to only and all heavy teenagers, except when used by food scientists, professionals who research what various foods do to and for people.

But when food scientists say that heavy teenagers are too heavy because of overeating, they're not finger-pointing or name-calling or character-bashing; they're not equating overeating with gluttony. Instead they are saying that heavy teenagers are too heavy because of accumulating too much unused food energy. We'll talk later about what this means and how it can happen.

IF YOU'RE TOO HEAVY IS IT BECAUSE YOU DON'T HAVE WILLPOWER?

Short answer: WILLPOWER DOESN'T EXPLAIN

At 14, obese and desperately wanting not to be obese, I began cutting down on pies, cakes, candy, fries, and the like. One evening, my grandfather, a physician, noticed that I had just refused my grandmother's rich unbelievably tasty homemade after dinner treat, which he knew I loved. Everybody loved it. He said admiringly, "Michael, you've got willpower." I was proud. Had I accepted the desert-offer, however, he instead might have scolded me saying your willpower battery needs a boost, and I would have felt bad.

Pointing to willpower deficiencies to explain why some people do things they shouldn't do and don't do things they should do attacks character. That's all willpower deficiency explanations can do. They don't tell you much of anything helpful. Even if I did lack willpower, this deficiency would not, could not, explain what made me and kept me too heavy. Some people talk as if it could, but it can't. The willpower analysis of overweight and obesity is hollow, heavy-handed, and circular. It goes like this: *if you're too heavy, you lack willpower, and the proof you do is you're too heavy.* Such reasoning travels round and round like a merry go round.

It's circular. It's cotton candy—looks substantial but is mostly air.

Maybe you find it hard to say no to anything sweet or fried. Maybe you find it hard to say yes to less TV, less computer time, and more exercise. But if all I know about you is that you are too heavy, I don't know if you have much, little, or no willpower. I know nothing of your strengths, weaknesses, or character.

WHY ARE HEAVY TEENS BULLIED AND TEASED?

Short answer: SOCIETY BLAMES THEM FOR IT

Pit bulls love meat, bullies love differences. And like the angry dog, the bully fixes on and tears at its prey, assuming without questioning or caring that heavy teenagers deserve it. After all, rationalizes the bully, it's their fault they're heavy. So it's okay to tease, ridicule, and torment them. Others watching won't mind, thinks the bully. Maybe they'll be glad. Maybe they'll join in."So the bully keeps on tormenting, ignoring the damage, hardship, and pain inflicted and disregarding the reasons that teenagers become heavy that aren't easily controlled. Bullies have too much fun ridiculing to let a little sympathy and understanding get in the way.

Our society may think weight-bullying is wrong, but it seems to okay the weight-prejudice that this kind of bullying feeds on. Such prejudice, aptly called the last frontier of socially accepted discrimination, is everywhere: in newspapers and magazines that promote thinness and demote heaviness; on television and in movies that rarely star obese or overweight actors; in doctors' offices with some doctors suggesting to or actually telling their heavy patients, "You're too heavy because you're too weak."

Weight-prejudice is often why some heavy job applicants aren't hired. It's even why some teachers treat heavy students as if lazy and incapable or as if different from the rest of the class. I remember feeling apart from everyone else when my first-grade teacher told the other boys and girls, "He (meaning me) should be our class Santa this year because he has more meat on his bones." I was honored to be the Santa, but confused and a little embarrassed by it as well. Why I was to be the chosen one bothered me, even at the tender age of six.

I know that from the fourth through the 12th grade I was a heavyweight; must have been one in the first grade, too.

15

WHAT'S BEING DONE TO STOP WEIGHT-BULLYING?

Short answer: RESEARCH CONTINUES

Putdowns discourage. When bullied about their weight—shamed and shunned for being too heavy—some teenagers get angry. Others get sad. Still others, particularly those teased about being heavy may eat excessively—binge eat—and gain more weight; actually, some teenagers even if not heavy will binge eat if made the butt of weight jokes.

Weight-bullying in all its forms has to stop, but how can we stop it? Unfortunately, there are no proven ways today, but perhaps there will be tomorrow. Here are a few promising ideas:

1. *Don't blame me.* As said, some weight-bullies justify what they do by blaming heavy teenagers for being heavy. The bully says it's your fault and so you deserve what you get from me. But no one deserves to be made fun of, no matter what. And, with respect to the finger-pointing and blaming, there's a lot of evidence to show that becoming and staying too heavy is often beyond one's control. So maybe by learning that blaming is unjustified, some weight bullies will see that shaming is illogical. That's the hope, anyway. To see if she could do it, that is convince a few hundred anti-overweight first-year college students that they might be wrong about the your-weight-is-your-fault idea, one of my graduate students taught this group of men and women some of the truths about overweight and obesity. It worked. The students became less prejudiced towards the heavy, but we don't know for how long the changes lasted.

2. *Others see it differently.* Would anti-overweight, anti-obese people become more understanding and less prejudiced towards the heavy if they thought others, people like their

own friends for instance, were? The idea, called **social consensus**, is if you think others similar to you don't share your beliefs, you'll change your beliefs to be more like theirs. It works when trying to reduce racial bigotry and sometimes when trying to reduce weight bigotry, too.

3. *Empathy — feeling the way it feels to feel the way.* Remember Sesame Street? If so, you surely recall Kermit the frog and his famous lament, "It's not easy being green." When the friendly frog said that, did he get your sympathy? More important, did he get your empathy? If sympathetic, you felt sad for him. If empathetic, not only did you feel sad for him you also understood his pain, the pain of feeling unlike those you long to be like. Perhaps teaching weight-bullies about how it feels to be heavy would help the bullies become more considerate, less prejudiced, and less ridiculing. Another of my graduate students is studying this promising idea.

Tomorrow's psychology may well change the hearts and minds of weight-bullies to improve the lives of heavy teens. But what can be done today?

WHAT CAN I DO NOW TO STOP BEING BULLIED ABOUT MY WEIGHT?

Short answer: TALK BACK ASSERTIVELY...WHEN POSSIBLE

If you're being bullied today, you want solutions today. Here's something to try. First, convince yourself that no one has the right to violate your rights, that no one has the right to tease or ridicule you for being heavy. Second, stand up for your rights by talking back assertively to the person trying to trample them.

For example, suppose you (somewhat on the heavy side) are at the dining room table with your four cousins, Aunt Barbara, and Uncle Mark. Mark's nice but has the sensitivity of an angry rhino. Dessert, a tray of nut squares, has just been placed on the table, and he loudly warns,

"Alana (*that's you*), better wait til everyone else has taken theirs. Don't know if we can trust you around all these sweets."

He grins. Everyone but you laughs.

How do you respond to Uncle Mark's ridicule? There are three choices, three ways: passively, aggressively (I don't recommend either), or assertively.

- *The passive way.* It skirts trouble. Say nothing or meekly say a few words with your eyes downcast and posture slumped, or, like others at the table, laugh. Basically, the passive response is just keep quiet. If you want things to improve, don't respond passively.

- *The aggressive way.* It provokes trouble. It clobbers feelings, invites retaliation, and brings out everyone's worst. Letting off steam may pump you up, but it likely angers and alienates the other person. If you want to be treated better, don't respond aggressively.

- *The assertive way.* It can end the problem without causing further trouble. It's not passive, because you speak up. It's not aggressive, because you speak well and don't trample feelings. To respond assertively to Uncle Mark, wait until he's alone and possibly say something like:

"Uncle Mark, I feel hurt and embarrassed by what happened tonight at dinner. My weight is personal to me, not a laughing matter. We have known and liked each other a long time, so please respect me and how I feel. I don't want to be teased or ridiculed about the way I am. Don't deserve it. OK?"

Suggestions for speaking assertively:

- speak respectfully, clearly, honestly, friendly, competently, considerately, and calmly.

- speak eye-to-eye.

- use lots of "I" statements (your feelings) and few "you" statements (accusations of "you did this" and "you did that").

Before trying out assertiveness on a weight bully, practice assertiveness. Practice alone in front of a mirror. Then practice with a special friend who fakes being the weight-bully while you play you. Practice like this until you're comfortable being assertive, and then trade places— now you play the bully and have your friend play you. By trading places, you'll get an idea of how weight bullies feel when talked to assertively.

ASSERTIVE TALK IS NOT THE REMEDY FOR ALL WEIGHT BULLYING. AVOID BULLIES WHO WOULD TEASE MORE OR GET PHYSICALLY ABUSIVE IF RESPONDED TO ASSERTIVELY.

Tell school authorities about them and get support from family and friends for doing so.

Two more things. First, as said, every time you're teased, ridiculed, or joked about for being heavy, tell yourself that no one has the right to do that. Second, before trying to talk assertively make sure you aren't angry, because sounding angry pushes others away. So, keep your cool. If you've lost it, get it back by breathing with your diaphragm while practicing breathing relaxation. The diaphragm is just below the lungs. Breathing with your diaphragm is like breathing when asleep:

a. Breathe-in and your stomach fills with air. (Put your hand on it, and you'll feel your hand move up.)

b. Breathe- out and your stomach flattens. (If still on your stomach, your hand will move back down.)

Master diaphragm breathing and then practice one of these two breathing-relaxation methods:

Breath-counting

1. Close your mouth.

2. Breathe-in slowly through your nose while counting from one to six or, if more comfortable, three.

3. Then, breathe-out slowly through your nose while counting the same way.

Breath-holding

1. Breathe-in through your nose, and hold your breath while counting from one to three.

2. Then, breathe-out through your mouth with your lips lightly pressed together, and softly say 'relax'. Repeat the breath-holding technique for several minutes.

Keep trying one of these breathing-better methods until you've calmed down.

~~

Teenage overweight and obesity are puzzles with many parts, as you'll see next.

Chapter 2:
Food Energy, Weight, and Me

Why do some teenagers gain weight faster than they should and yet others, even some who eat like there was no tomorrow, don't? Are calories really little evildoers in food? What's the difference between energy and energetic and between potential and actual energy? How can too much energy make you heavy? How can burning up something make it work? Do people get heavy because of their calorie consumption or because of their genes or because of their family? How are a log and a loaf of bread alike? You'll be able to answer questions like these after reading this chapter. They touch upon critical parts of the puzzle of being too heavy.

WHAT IS FOOD ENERGY?

Short answer: FUEL

Food supplies food energy, energy needed to stay alive. An ample diet will always be your source of food energy—fuel for you—doing for you what car fuel does for the car: making everything work. Car fuel (gasoline or electricity or both) runs the car—no fuel, no energy, no go. Body fuel (food energy) runs you —no fuel, no energy, no go...no life.

DOES FOOD ENERGY MAKE YOU ENERGETIC?

Short answer: MAYBE, ESPECIALLY IF IT COMES FROM NUTRITIOUS FOODS

Eat a dinner of spaghetti and meatballs, and you've supplied yourself with a large amount of food energy. After finishing the meal, will you feel *energetic*—strong, peppy, ready to do homework, able to play an hour of basketball, able to run two miles? Will all that energy give you what you need to successfully carry on the next few hours of your day, to enjoy its pleasures and face its challenges? Quite likely it will, depending on how physically fit you are and if things are going reasonably well in your life.

But suppose during dinner you have an argument with your parents or find out someone you care for has rejected you or learn that the term paper you had struggled to turn in on time was worth only a "D". Depressing events like these can suck the energy from your body and, for a while at least, leave you as weak as a sparrow flying into a headwind; that's the opposite of feeling energetic. Events sending your mood into a tailspin will sap your feelings of strength, no matter how well and how much you eat—no matter how nutritious and plentiful your diet.

Yet, rest assured that eating well will, in the long run, serve you well, giving you the energy needed to stay strong, healthy, and alive and to feel and be energetic.

HOW DO YOU FIND OUT HOW MUCH FOOD ENERGY A FOOD HAS?

Short answer: BURN IT AND SEE HOW HOT IT GETS

Different foods in different amounts provide different amounts of food energy. For instance, 10 ounces of steak provides more food energy than 5 ounces of it does and both more than 30 ounces of lettuce will. To determine how much energy a particular food is capable of providing, scientists will first set the food on fire and then, as it burns, find out how much heat it creates—more heat, more energy. The amount of heat, energy, is measured in calorie-units.

A calorie of energy is a unit of heat, just like a pound is a unit of weight and an inch is a unit of height. The hotter the food gets the higher the number of calories of energy it is said to have. Actually, when food scientists talk about calories of energy, they're really not talking about something as tiny as a calorie. They're talking about an amount of energy 1000 times bigger called a *kilocalorie*. One kilocalorie (kcal) is the heat needed to raise one kilogram of water one degree centigrade.

Because most people mean kilocalories when they say calories, we'll do that, too; in this book, we'll use the two terms interchangeably. We'll also, as do many, talk of calories as if they were little things in food. But of course they are not that at all. They're just units of food energy: the amount of fuel the food is capable of giving you.

That fuel, coming from the food you eat, is made available once you digest the food. Here's a silly question: What is an apple before you eat and digest it? The answer: an apple. Or, more to the point I want to make about energy, an apple is a piece of fruit with *potential* energy. Here's another silly question: what's a log in a fireplace before you set the log on fire? The answer: a piece of wood with *potential* energy.

A log usually smells good in the fireplace, but you'll get no warmth from the log by just smelling it or seeing it. For the log's *potential* energy to become **actual** energy that will warm you, the log must burn. Burning is the key that unlocks the log's warming power.

The same goes for food. It gives us energy, but not by just seeing or smelling it, or even by chewing and swallowing it. To convert its *potential* energy into *actual* energy, your body must break down the food inside you into a substance that can get into your bloodstream. That process of breaking down the food is digestion, and like burning the log in the fireplace, it's the key that unlocks the food's energy.

WHAT DO YOU USE THE FOOD ENERGY FOR?

Short answer: LIVING AND THRIVING

You spend your food energy, the largest part of it anyway, just to stay alive—breathing, pumping blood, growing, etc.. Usually you don't know you're spending it like this when you are, even though these life-preserving tasks dig way into your supply of calories. You also spend calories of food energy every day doing things like lifting, running, walking, playing, napping, taking out the garbage, talking on the phone, showering, and more. These calorie-burners you're usually quite aware of doing.

So, to live and thrive— to meet your needs and wants— you require many calories of food energy minute by minute, day by day throughout your life. But how do you know how many calories of it you need and the essential food groups to get it from? One way is to visit Choosemyplate, a website will talk about later.

HOW DO YOU BECOME TOO HEAVY?

Short answer: TOO MUCH UNUSED FOOD ENERGY PILES-UP

We just said that for you to keep going and doing what you need and want to do requires many calories of food energy every day. But, we should add, *not too many of them*. Definitely not more than you can use up in a reasonable amount of time. Calories are meant to be spent. That's because what your body doesn't use up, piles up, creating a surplus of unused, left over, calories of food energy. If day after day, week after week, and month after month, the surplus gets bigger and bigger, your body will eventually put it into storage, and you'll gain weight.

An adult gains about a pound or so of fat every time his or her body stores approximately 3500 surplus calories of leftover, unused, food energy.

WHY DOES THE CALORIE SURPLUS FORM, WHAT MAKES IT HAPPEN?

Short answer: TOO MUCH EATING, TOO LITTLE MOVING, OR BOTH

To understand how and why a calorie surplus (energy surplus) forms, imagine the scale in the picture is an energy scale with two trays.

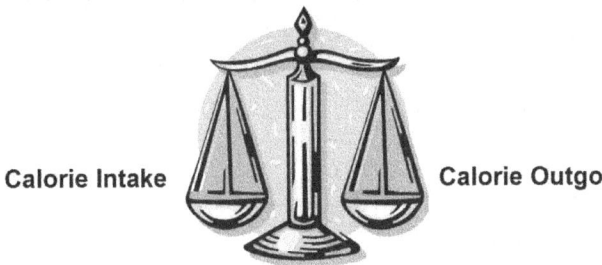

Calorie Intake   Calorie Outgo

On the left hangs the calorie intake tray. It stands for the calories of food energy you get from what you eat after digestion. On the right hangs the calorie outgo tray. It stands for the calories of food energy you spend, as said, staying alive and healthy and doing the things you want to do.

When you get as many calories as you spend, the two trays of the energy scale are, as pictured, balanced; there's no surplus of leftover calories to form—**calorie intake = calorie outgo.**

What if, however, you use up more calories than you bring in and the intake of calories no longer equals the outgo of them? The trays would no longer be balanced, but in this situation there still wouldn't be a calorie surplus. Instead, there would be a calorie deficit, meaning that you've spent more calories than you've acquired—**calorie outgo >calorie intake**. When calorie deficits are large and lasting, weight is lost.

Now let's suppose that for a long time instead of spending more calories of food energy than you acquire you acquire more than you spend. Maybe you have eaten too many rich foods each day or have been idle too much of the time, or maybe and most likely you have done both: eaten too much and exercised too little. The result is the same: **calorie intake >calorie outgo**. Regardless of the reasons you've taken in more calories than you've used up, a calorie surplus would form, and the calorie intake tray would hang lower than the calorie outgo one.

It's desirable, healthy, and essential for growing teenagers to get lots of good quality food energy every day. But it's neither desirable nor healthy, let alone essential, for them to have so much food energy left over for days on end that they gain too much weight.

HOW COME SOME TEENAGERS CAN EAT EVERYTHING AND ANYTHING AND NOT GET TOO HEAVY?

Short answer: INEFFICIENCY

I know a fellow who eats at least five times a day. He calls himself a junkfood junkie because much of what he eats is drive through-fast food and snacks like cheese covered crackers, candy, and cola. He eats nutritiously at times, but prefers the junkfood. It's a mainstay of his life, has been for years. He exercises, but not all that much, yet is and has always been as thin as a rail. I don't envy him, because the way he eats is not the road to good health, but that he eats as he does without exercising for hours a day yet still keeps his weight down intrigues me. One reason his weight doesn't mushroom out of control might be that his body isn't very efficient in the way it deals with food, certainly it's not as efficient as mine is; I gain weight quite easily.

Efficient bodies, like mine, are expert energy-hunters. They capture lots of calories of energy from the foods they digest and so have lots of calories available to spend. Yet they're stingy energy-spenders.

To see the difference between efficient and somewhat inefficient bodies, consider what might happen if my junkfood-loving friend, call him Dave, and I each were to treat ourselves to equally huge helpings of chocolate cake topped with equally ample portions of vanilla ice cream. I possibly could get 1200 calories of food energy from the splurge, whereas Dave might get only 800 calories from it. Suppose that awhile after enjoying the rich foods, we play an hour of tennis, walk back to our offices about a mile away, read two hours, and talk on the phone for one more hour. Of course during this entire time we've been breathing and doing all the other essential jobs of staying alive. Let's say the cost of all these activities for me is 800 calories of energy, leaving me with 400 calories left over from the 1200 calorie treat. The cost of them for Dave is 1000 calories of energy. So he has no calories left over; actually he has spent more calories than he has obtained from the cake à la mode.

The following table shows the calories-in and calories-out score for Dave and me, both of us eating the same kind and amount of food and doing the same kind and amount of activity:

	Efficient me	Not so efficient Dave
Calories acquired	1200	800
Calories spent	800	1000
Calories left over	400	(-200)

So it seems that my body is more efficient than my friend Dave's. I was able to harness more of the foods' calories and spend fewer of them, even though in no way did we differ from one another in what we ate or did afterwards. If calories were dollars, I'd be richer than my pal.

But would I be luckier? Well, it depends. If there's a drought causing a long food shortage, and Dave and I go hungry for many days, I'm the luckier one. My efficient body will get through the ordeal better than his will. I'll get more precious calories of food energy from what little food I do find and spend less of them to keep going.

Genes for this kind of efficiency, some scientists believe, developed eons ago during prehistoric times when periods of famine (no food) alternated with periods of feasting (lots of food). The cave-dwellers with the efficiency genes compared with those without them had a great advantage. They were able to get lots of calories from the foods they ate during the times of feasting and more calories from the foods they managed to find during the times of famine. The larger reserves of food energy they were therefore able to build up would enable them, in comparison with cave dwellers without efficiency genes, to stay alive longer. Those folks who didn't have them could not as easily acquire the needed supply of life-saving energy and so would be more likely to starve to death.

No one knows for certain if this theory of efficiency-genes and how they came to be is true, but it is plausible. What is certain, however, is that without enough food energy, the body won't survive. So, when droughts, wars, or other catastrophes make food scarce, one needs a body that has been and continues to be good at milking the energy out of food and stingy when spending it. If there's not much food to go around, one needs an efficient body, like mine is.

But what if there's plenty of food available and famines don't happen for most of us? What if supermarkets, restaurants,

28

convenience stores, and well-stocked refrigerators are everywhere for just about everyone? Then, few of us will need or want a body that's very efficient. Such a body would absorb too many calories of energy and spend too few of them for too long and so would too easily gain and hold onto unwanted pounds. If you're lucky enough to live where there's plenty to eat and get plenty to eat, you're better off having a somewhat inefficient body, like Dave's.

Teenagers with them spend lots of calories just living, let alone working and playing, and seem able to eat nearly anything and everything, yet stay slim.

WILL MY GENES CAUSE ME TO BE TOO HEAVY?

Short answer: RARELY WITHOUT YOUR HELP

If the theory about efficiency genes is true, then perhaps some of us will have a harder time not becoming overweight or obese. But the theory is only a theory and doesn't explain all the reasons for weight problems. It also doesn't explain how genes work.

You were born after developing trillions of cells each with 46 chromosomes—23 from each parent, 23 pairs. The chromosomes carry the hundreds to thousands of genes making you, you. Some genes affect you now, others will affect you later on. Some genes—you've approximately 20,000-25,000 of them— determine whether you're a blonde, brunette, or redhead. Others say whether you have blue eyes, hazel eyes, or brown eyes and still others whether you have black, red, white, or brown skin. You can make these features *appear* different without actually changing them: wear contact lenses so your naturally brown eyes *appear* to be blue; apply dye so your naturally brunette hair *appears* to be red; spread on lotions and creams so your naturally light skin *appears* to be dark. But all that you can do with the lenses, the dyes, and the creams is to artificially mask features, not really change them. They're still the same underneath the mask. What they truly are has been determined by your genes; genes rule here.

But not everywhere. Genes aren't so bossy with abilities and talents. What these eventually become is up to you. So, for instance, if you were born with a natural talent for the violin, you'll have to nurture that talent. You'll need to take lessons from a violin virtuoso and practice for hours every day for years before debuting at Carnegie Hall. Likewise, if you were born with a natural ability to run swiftly and tirelessly, you'll have to nurture that ability. You'll need instruction from a great coach and years of practice before competing at the Olympics. Genes don't rule here. They contribute to your talents and abilities, but you must perfect them.

Likewise, some genes may increase the chances of your having a weight problem in the same way that eating poorly increases your chances of getting sick. But rarely do genes alone make weight problems inevitable; your input is essential. In other words, of major importance in deciding whether or not you're going to be too heavy is what, how much, and how often you eat and how active a life you lead.

IS MY WEIGHT AFFECTED BY WHAT MY PARENTS WEIGH?

Short answer: SOMEWHAT

Generally, heaviness runs in families. If both your mom and dad are heavy, the chance you will be heavy is about 80%. Those odds drop-down to 40%, if only one of them weighs a lot and to just 10%, if neither does. As well, there's some evidence that the very heaviest mothers and fathers raise the very heaviest sons and daughters.

Even though such statements are based on carefully done scientific studies of thousands of families, they still only say what might happen not what will happen. What you weigh today and will weigh to tomorrow have more to do with your own eating and moving than with what your folks weigh.

~~

There are various parts to the overweight/obesity puzzle as you have seen. Exactly how they all fit together is not as yet completely understood. But what we do know is that being too heavy is a problem, as the next chapter describes.

Chapter 3:
The Problem

So what if teenagers are getting heavier? What's wrong with that?

Find out here.

ARE MANY TEENS TOO HEAVY?

Short answer: DEFINITELY

More teenagers today are overweight or obese than ever before. Sixteen of every hundred 12 to 19-year-olds has a weight problem. That's a greater percentage of young people than in the 1960s when about five of every hundred teens was too heavy and even more than in the 1990s and as late as 2002. Overweight and obesity are still on the upswing, in not only the USA but also other parts of the world.

What's even more alarming than the data on skyrocketing percentages of teenagers who weigh too much are the data on how heavy they are in fact becoming. Heavy teens are heavier than they have ever been.

WHAT'S AT STAKE IF YOU'RE TOO HEAVY?

Short answer: DISEASE, DISCOMFORT, DESPAIR NOW AND LATER

If too heavy now, you're at risk of having health and social problems now as well as in years to come. Let's look at tomorrow's threats first.

The future. If too heavy now, chances are you'll be too heavy when an adult. And carrying around those extra pounds then increases your risk of diseases including type 2 diabetes, cancer, and stroke. The risks worsen for those largest around their middles — the Apple- shapes.

Jake and Lorenzo are each 40 years-old, the same height and weight, and equally overweight. But although equally overweight, they differ in how they are overweight, that is in how their surplus pounds distribute on their bodies. Jake, for instance, is wider at the hips than at the waist. His 42 inch hips and 36 inch waist give him a kind of pear-shape. Lorenzo, in contrast, is wider at the waist than at the hips. His 42 inch waist and 36 inch hips make him more of an apple-shape. By dividing waist size by hip size, which is computing what's called the waist to hips ratio, a person can find out what his or her shape is mostly like. When a man's waist to hip ratio is greater than 1, he's an Apple, and when a woman's is .85 or more, she's also one. For both sexes, the apple shape is the most unhealthy and risky way to lug around one's fat. Even if Lorenzo were just 17 years-old instead of 40, his apple-shape would still be a bad omen.

The present. Heavy teenagers face three threats during their teenage years because of being heavy: discomfort, disease, despair. These are the three D's of being a teenager who's too heavy.

About the first two, some overweight or obese boys and girls find playing sports and even walking hard to do because of joint pain, excessive sweating, and difficulty breathing. Others may experience worse things like type II diabetes, high blood pressure, and high cholesterol.

Yet as bad as discomfort and disease are, even more upsetting for many heavy teenagers is the despair they feel from the rejection and ridicule they experience and endure. Weight prejudice can make a heavy teenager's school years miserable, as the recollection that follows illustrates:

34

"Middle school was as bad as grade school. In both the kids who hated fat kids were everywhere. In eighth grade I was 5 feet tall and 170 pounds and teased, teased, teased. So for relief, I watched lots of TV and snacked; I needed the escape.

If middle school was awful, high school was pure torture. One day during swimming class, the coach yelled, `Everybody out of the pool,' and like regimented troops everyone, except me, pulled up. I couldn't. The laughter was deafening. I laughed as loudly as the others did. What else could I do?

I can't explain why, but wrestling class was required for grade 10 boys. Like me, the teacher was obese, but unlike me was super-strong. He loved the powerful and hated the weak. He acted as if anyone who wasn't strong, especially if fat, was garbage, expendable. I fit perfectly into his category of, "you' re worthless." Maybe that's why this King Kong coach made me his 200 pound whipping boy to repeatedly demonstrate wrestling holds on. After a few weeks of this torture, I begged my doctor, who also was my grandfather, to get me out of all the gym classes. He did. (I'd had asthma years earlier.) His written excuse did end the wrestling class agony, but unfortunately cut off other sources of fitness I desperately needed.

Not everything in my life back then, however, was bleak. There was Jocelyn Ray who with her silky hair, brown eyes, full lips, porcelain skin, and curves was irresistible. I truly loved her. She sat a couple desks away from me in Geometry and like me hated it, but unlike me couldn't do the work. I silently vowed to save her, so mustering every ounce of courage (talking to a pretty girl turned me to rubber then), I volunteered to help. `Don't worry, I'll show you how to do this stuff.' We met at her house after school, and fearful but hopeful, butterflies fluttering in my stomach, I tutored her. During the two hours it took, I kept my stomach sucked in despite the discomfort of doing so and, by sitting across from her at all times, prevented her from seeing my rather large love handles. If she thought I was fat (she must have), she never let on. Jocelyn had class.

Being so near her at the kitchen table, I felt my love for her grow.

I offered further tutoring for the next day, but she said no thanks, adding that I'd already helped plenty and was 'wonderful for taking the time to.' Her kindness gave me hope that there could be more between us, yet her refusal of further lessons left me unsure.

That confusion vanished in a flash the next day, however. I saw her holding hands with handsome Harper Conner, a boy my age but 50 pounds lighter and 10 inches smaller in the waist. And, to my growing disgust, no love handles. I hated Harper Conner. Geometry class ended a few weeks later, and summer vacation began. Now I could hide out at home safe from the fat-hating world outside. I wasted my 15th summer snacking while watching TV all day, every day."

~~

Not every heavy teenager suffers discomfort, disease, or despair. But for those who do, there are ways to brighten their futures, as the healthy weight management chapters to follow show. First, however, let's look at how overweight and obesity are measured in the 21st-century.

CHAPTER 4
Too Heavy?

What does too heavy mean? Is overweight the same thing as obesity, and how is it the same or different? What's the best way to find out if you're too heavy? How do doctors and other health professionals find out if a teenager is too heavy? Lots of people talk about the body mass index. What is it, where did it come from, what's so good about it, how do you compute and interpret it, what should a teenager's body mass index be? Chapter 4 answers these and similar questions about being too heavy.

HOW DO I KNOW IF I'M TOO HEAVY?

Short answer: MEASURE AND INTERPRET YOUR BMI

If 16-year-old Ronny is heavier than his friends, maybe he's too heavy; but maybe he's not. If 13-year-old Arceda no longer fits into the new pants she wore last summer, maybe she's too heavy; but maybe she's not. If 17-year-old Al-Noor can pinch an inch around his middle, maybe he's too heavy; but maybe he's not.

To say if one of these teens, is too heavy, someone has to figure out that teenager's body mass index (BMI). Usually the someone doing that job is a doctor, dietitian, weight management specialist, school nurse, gym teacher, or guidance counselor. But teenagers can periodically and easily do this for themselves, as you'll see.

Who invented the BMI? In 1835, a math whiz living in Belgium named Adolphe Quetelet, developed the body mass index. Born in Ghent, Belgium in 1796 and dying in 1874, Quetelet was one of the great scientists of his time. His work on the body mass index, however, didn't take the world by storm right away. In fact, 150 years passed before scientists and doctors caught onto its value. Today most health care workers rely on it in their struggles against teenage overweight and obesity.

What's the BMI used for? Doctors and other health professionals use the BMI to locate the teenagers at risk of getting a life-altering disease. To professionals concerned about the health and well-being of teenagers, finding a large BMI is seeing a flashing red light signaling danger ahead.

What's the BMI and what does it mean? The BMI measures how heavy a person is in relation to how tall that person is. With some extra things thrown in, the BMI is simply weight divided by height. Generally, a shorter heavier adult will have a larger body mass index than a taller lighter adult. When an adult's BMI is at or between 25 and 29.9, that person is overweight and when it's 30 or more, obese. Sex and age don't matter; these BMI values apply to all adults.

Sex and age do matter, however, when the person in question is a child or adolescent. As the Centers for Disease Control and Prevention (CDC) points out, typical levels of body fat change with age and gender, significantly so among children and teens. To say if a particular teenager's BMI indicates that he or she is too heavy, we have to find out how it compares with the BMI of others that teenager's age and sex — that teenager's reference group. So, Ronny's BMI would be compared with the body mass indexes of his reference group (other 16 year-old boys). Likewise, Arceda's BMI would be compared with those of her reference group (other 13-year-old girls) and Al-Noor's with those of his. Any teenager whose body mass index is larger than those of most of that teenager's reference group is too heavy. But how much larger is too much larger?

WHEN IS A TEENAGER OBESE?

Short answer: BMI AT OR ABOVE THE 95TH PERCENTILE OF REFERENCE GROUP

Teenagers are obese when at least 95% of their reference group (others their age and sex) have a lower body mass index.

So, for 13-year-old Arceda to be considered obese, at least 95% of other 13-year-old girls must have a BMI that's not as large as hers. Think of it this way. Suppose you build many huge hotels with many huge rooms, all told, enough space for all girls Arceda's age in America to live. In each available room you put 100 of these 13-year-old girls. Some of them will be taller than Arceda, and some will be shorter. All will be her age, however. Yet, Arceda's BMI is at or above the 95th percentile of her reference group. So her BMI will be greater than those of at least 95 out of 100 girls in nearly every room.

Obesity is having a BMI at or above the 95th percentile of one's reference group.

WHEN IS A TEENAGER OVERWEIGHT?

Short answer: BMI AT OR BETWEEN 85TH & 95TH PERCENTILES OF REFERENCE GROUP

Overweight is just a step away from obesity. The overweight teenager's BMI is less than the 95th percentile but at or above the 85th percentile of his or her reference group. Too heavy is, as said, being either obese or overweight.

The CDC has BMI information on thousands of US residents and so is able to chart their year by year BMI changes. The table that follows shows the BMI cutoffs for 12 to 19-year-old boys and girls that the CDC says indicates obesity or overweight.

BMI's FOR TEENAGERS
OBESITY (OB) & OVERWEIGHT (OW)

	BOYS		GIRLS	
Age	OB	OW	OB	OW
12	24.2	21.0-24.1	25.2	21.6-25.1
13	25.1	21.8- 25	26.2	22.6-26.1
14	26.0	22.6-25.9	27.2	23.4-27.1
15	26.8	23.4-26.7	28.0	24.0-27.9
16	27.6	24.2-27.5	28. 8	24.6-28.7
17	28.2	24.7-28.1	29.6	25.2-29.5
18	28.9	25.6-28.8	30.2	25.6-30.1
19	29.6	26.4-29.5	31.0	26.1-30.9

A BMI in the **obesity** (OB) column signifies being at or greater than the 95th percentile. For example, a girl of 15 with a BMI=28 is obese; at least 95% of the other 15-year-old girls in her reference group have a BMI that's less than hers.

A BMI in the **overweight** (OW) column signifies being at or greater than the 85th percentile but less than the 95th percentile. For example, a boy of 15 with a BMI at or between 23.4-26.7 is considered to be overweight.

Source: CDC body mass index-for-age percentiles for boys 2 to 20 years and for girls 2 to 20 years. May 30, 2000

The CDC also says that normal weight is having a BMI between the 5th percentile and just under the 85th percentile of one's reference group, and underweight is having a BMI less than the 5th percentile.

HOW DO I CALCULATE MY BODY MASS INDEX (BMI) MYSELF?

There are two ways, metric and linear. Each gives the same answer and each relies on measuring height and weight accurately. The best scales, tall, solid, and heavy, are the types that doctors, school nurses, and many gym teachers employ; usually such scales come with attached rulers for measuring height. Use scales like these when computing your BMI, if at all possible.

Now, let's calculate the BMI of a 13-year-old 155 lb, 5 ft 4in (64 in) girl.

---

1. THE METRIC WAY TO CALCULATE THE BMI:

The metric formula for BMI is weight in kilograms divided by height in meters squared.

BMI = weight (in kilograms)/height2 (in meters).

(a) 155 pounds = 70.31 kg

(b) 5'4" (64 inches)=1.625 m.

(c) m2(1.625x 1.625) = 2.64m

BMI= 70.3 kg/2.64 m

BMI = 26.6

---

2. THE LINEAR WAY TO CALCULATE THE BMI.

Instead of kilograms and meters, this formula uses pounds and inches. You'll probably prefer it to the metric formula if you customarily think of weight in pounds and height in inches.

BMI =weight (in pounds) x 703/height 2 (in inches)

(a) linear formula multiplier for weight = 703

155 (lb) x 703 =108965lb

(b) height squared = 64in x 64in = 4096in

BMI = 10,8965lb/4096in = 26.6

A 13-year-old girl whose BMI = 26.6 is above the 95th percentile of her reference group and so is considered likely to be obese.

HOW DO I TRACK MY BODY MASS INDEX ONLINE?

Short answer: GO TO THE CDC WEBSITE

To keep track of your BMI online, periodically visit the Center for Disease Control BMI calculator webpage at: http://apps.nccd.cdc.gov/dnpabmi/Calculator.aspx.

There you'll see a Calculator box for entering information about yourself that this online site needs to compute and interpret your BMI. If online now, go to this webpage. Let's say you're a 5'8", 15-year-old boy who weighs 213 lbs. You were born February 13, 1995, and today it's March 10, 2010. Enter all this information in the box on the webpage:

BMI CALCULATOR BOX

1. Birth Date: February 13 1995

2. Date of Measurement: March 10, 2010

3. Sex: Boy (x) Girl

4. Height: 5 feet 8 inches

5. Weight to nearest 1/4 pound: 213 pounds

Adapted from Division of Nutrition, Physical Activity, and Obesity National Center for Chronic Disease Prevention and Health Promotion

After finishing, click the calculate button and a new page will pop up that computes and interprets your BMI. It will say that your BMI is 32.4, which is too high for 15-year-old boys because it's at the 98th percentile of their reference group. Also, there will be a warning of possible obesity and related health problems and advice to see a doctor.

DOES YOUR BODY MASS INDEX (BMI) TELL YOU HOW FAT YOU ARE?

Short answer: NO

We all have fat. When you were just a cuddly newborn, about 12% of you was fat. The fat was housed as triglyceride (the main kind of fat the body stores) in five to six billion special cells called fat-cells. By the time you took your first steps, you likely were twice as fat as during those beginning few weeks, but later on, without trying to, probably slimmed-down. Suppose now, however, that you're 32% fat. If so, chances are you have billions and billions and billions of fat-cells and are too heavy.

43

The BMI will say if you're too heavy, and because it's a fairly reliable sign of fatness — better than weight alone is — if you may be too fat. But it can't say how fat you are, meaning how much fat you have on your body. And it can't say if others your age and sex with a BMI the same as yours have as much, more, or less fat on them than you.

Weight and fat are different things. Let's say Mary weighs 100 pounds. Essentially that 100 pounds comprises the non-fat part of Mary (muscle, bone, blood, water) and the fat part of her. Suppose Mary is 20% fat. That means 20 pounds or 20% of her 100 pounds is fat, and 80 pounds or 80% of it is everything else. But from just stepping on a weight scale Mary will never know how much of her is fat and how much isn't. She'll only know her weight, and weight by itself doesn't say all that much about fat.

In fact, it's possible for one person to be fatter than another even though both individuals are the same sex, age, height, and weight. For instance, consider two 17-year-old boys, each of whom weighs 175 pounds and stands 5'10". One plays hockey in winter, soccer in spring, and football in fall. As well, he swims in summer and, no matter what the season, loves to run. He's a mover. The other 175 pound teen also loves sports, but he'd rather watch them played, not play them. He avoids contact sports, seeks spectator sports, and almost never swims or runs. He's a sitter, mostly.

Because the boys are the same weight and height, their body mass indexes are equal — BMI for each boy =25.1. That puts them, according to the BMI cutoffs for 17 year-old boys (see above), over the 85th percentile but under the 95th percentile of their reference group, so they're both classified as overweight. But compared with the mover, the sitter is probably fatter. The less active boy likely has a larger waist, smaller forearms and biceps, and less muscular legs than the more active boy. In other words, chances are that more of the sitter's 175 pounds compared with the mover's 175 pounds consists of fat. The BMI alone can't reveal with any degree of certainty which boy is the fatter or by how much. One way to find out, however, would be to compare the boys' skinfolds.

Skinfold measurement will tell the doctor more than the BMI will about how fat someone is. When health professionals measure skinfolds, they pinch specific parts of the body, like the triceps muscle at the back of the arm. They do so to assess how much of what's pinched comprises fat tissue. Special scissor-like precisely calibrated devices called skinfold calipers are used for the pinching, which by the way doesn't hurt.

~~

TOO HEAVY MEANS OVERWEIGHT OR OBESE, but overweight isn't exactly the same thing as obese. Technically, overweight means excess weight, and obesity means excess fat.

Chapter 5
Concerns

What worries you about taking charge of your BMI? Is it giving up things you don't want to give up? Is it not knowing who is there to help you? Is it not understanding what to aim for? This chapter answers several major concerns that teenagers considering the pros and cons weight management express.

DO I HAVE TO GIVE UP TV AND VIDEO GAMES?

Short answer: NO

No need to stop watching TV or to stop playing videos. They're fun, relaxing, and renewing. But so are tennis, swimming, racquetball, baseball, lifting weights, running, and more; plus, sports and other vigorous activities like them will help manage your weight.

How much awake time do you spend sitting or lying down, and how much on the go? To find out, record what you do each day for a week. Keep tabs on the minutes spent moving and on those used up not moving. No need to be exact, just try to record what's happening as it happens. To do that well, divide a piece of paper lengthwise and designate one column for minutes of sitting or lying down and the other for minutes of moving. The results at the end of the week may shock you.

Move more, as later chapters advise. Work up to at least 60 minutes of vigorous activity each day. There'll still be plenty of time for TV and the computer.

SHOULD I STAY AWAY FROM PARTIES WHERE THERE'S LOTS OF FOOD?

Short answer: NO

Food isn't your enemy; denial is. If you feel too deprived while on the road to a healthier weight, you'll likely also feel cheated and robbed, and as a result detour from your path or quit the trip altogether. So, don't deny yourself a party because the good food there will tempt you; occasional treats are part of healthy weight management.

Most important, don't create lists of forbidden foods and couple them with *never again promises,* such as

- "Never again will my lips touch another doughnut," (but you love doughnuts).

- "Never again will I snack while watching TV," (but the escape feels great).

- "Never again will I go to Burger Palace and eat fries," (but all your friends go there and have them).

- "Never again will I eat birthday cake," (but you love birthday parties and would hate going and then refusing the cake).

Undoubtedly, you will sometimes have a doughnut and sometimes have birthday cake and sometimes snack while enjoying TV and sometimes go with your friends after school to a fast food restaurant. *Never again promises* never last.

So don't make them, you'll only break them. Worse than breaking them is feeling so bad for having done so that you call yourself weak and hopeless. Avoid never again promises and the all or nothing thinking (*either I always eat it or I never eat it*) underlying them. Manage your weight without confusing healthy moderation with unhealthy, unrealistic, and unnecessary self-denial.

48

SHOULD I COUNT CALORIES?

Short answer: NOT IF YOU'LL OBSESS OVER THEM

Count them to shop smarter. Let's say the label on a packaged food you're considering indicates that it possesses 1700 cal of food energy and weighs 300 g. Reading more of the label, you see that each nutrient in this food weighs 100 g: 100 g of protein, 100 g of carbohydrate, and 100 g of fat. But does that mean that the three nutrients provide equivalent amounts of energy? No. Fat provides more than twice the calories, gram for gram, than either protein or carbohydrate does.

- 1 g of protein provides about 4 cal, so, 100 g = about 400 cal

- 1 g carbohydrate provides about 4 cal, so, 100 g = about 400 cal

- 1 g fat provides over 9 cal, so, 100 g = over 900 cal

So, this 1700 calorie packaged food is definitely a high-fat food: over 900 of its 1700 calories are from fat. Maybe knowing it is so high in that ingredient will stop you from buying it. Again, count calories to shop smarter.

Relatedly, count them to compare foods and discover the nutritional bargains among them. Nutritional bargains, like fruits and vegetables, provide the best nutrition for each calorie of energy that the food makes available. Calorie for calorie, nutritional bargains are good deals. Two hundred grams of sliced apple, for instance, has fewer calories, and more nutrition—and appeases hunger better—than a 200 g slice of apple pie loaded with refined sugar. Nutritional bargains promote healthier living.

So used wisely, calorie knowledge can help you. Used unwisely, however, it can do just the opposite. One misuse of calorie knowledge is calorie obsession. To explain, some teenagers worry to the point of obsession that they'll have too many calories unless they eat only foods that claim to be low in them or diet so ruthlessly that they almost starve themselves. But choosing foods based only on their calorie amounts without considering their nutritional value, or dieting just to escape calories are recipes for becoming weak, tired, and sick. Worst of all, counting calories as if the Count on Sesame Street — preoccupied, almost hypnotized by the numbers — steps towards developing an eating disorder.

SHOULD I COUNT CARBOHYDRATES (CARBS)?

Short answer: ONLY IF A DOCTOR OR DIETITIAN ADVISES YOU TO

The best reason to count carbohydrates is to ensure getting an ample supply of them; we all need carbohydrate daily. Those who try to cut way down on this nutrient are usually adults on a high fat, high protein diet that demands carbohydrate restriction. Not a good plan for growing teenagers. Without enough carbohydrate they can't sufficiently break down the fat in their foods which causes fat fragments known as ketone bodies to build up. Ketosis, a condition resulting from this build up, leads to various problems not the worst of which is embarrassingly horrid breath.

Unless directed to by a doctor or dietitian, teenagers should never severely curtail their carbohydrate intake.

WHO SHOULD I ASK TO HELP ME?

Short answer: A DOCTOR, OTHER PROFESSIONALS, YOUR FAMILY

Talk with your family doctor if you think you're too heavy. As said, she or he will determine if the concern is justified; it may not be. If you are too heavy, however, the doctor will tell you what to do about it, including if necessary, to see a dietitian or psychologist specializing in weight management. Talk as well with your parents. Ask them to buy nutritious snack foods and create meals that assist your weight management efforts. Also, if feasible, seek the support of brothers, sisters, uncles, aunts, grandparents, special friends, the school guidance counselor, and the school nurse.

Get help. Support fosters success. So, as you pursue a healthier weight, encourage others to help you financially, educationally, behaviorally, emotionally. Don't bear the weight management burden alone.

WHAT SHOULD MY GOAL BE?

Short answer: TO LOWER YOUR BMI

If an adult and overweight or obese, your goal would be to lose weight so your BMI would decrease. How much you'd need to lose to reach a healthier BMI would depend on how heavy you were. However, you're a teenager, and that changes the rules. If overweight or obese, your task like the adult's is still to lower your BMI. But, unlike the adult, you might be able to do that without losing any weight whatsoever. In fact, if you have a lot of growing yet to do, lowering your BMI without losing weight may be exactly what you should do.

There are three ways to change the BMI: slowing down the speed of gaining, stopping the gaining altogether, and losing weight. Your doctor knows which of them is best for you.

Slowing down. It's expected that growing teenagers will gain weight. That's normal. But if putting on the pounds too fast, they'll either have to stop gaining for a time or slow it down to bring their BMI into line with the BMI of others their age and sex. The doctor is likely to prescribe slowing down for mildly to moderately heavy teenagers with a fair amount of growing still to do.

51

Slowing down is a most effective way to reach a healthier weight without losing any weight at all. Consider, for instance, a 5'6", 17-year-old boy who weighs 160 pounds and has a BMI = 25.8. He's overweight, according to the standards named earlier, because 89% of all other 17 year-old boys have a BMI that's lower than 25.8. Suppose that for the next 10 months, with the help of his doctor, he's able to reduce the speed that he has previously been gaining. Now, 10 months later, he's not only 10 months older but also 3 inches taller and 3 pounds heavier. So, his BMI is 24.1, which means he's no longer overweight. In other words, because he's older, taller, and not too much heavier than he was 10 months earlier, his BMI has decreased enough — from 25.8 to 24.1 — for him to be out of the overweight category. Instead of 89% of the other teens in his reference group having a lower BMI, only 75% of them do. The boy was able to lose overweight without losing any weight at all and reach a healthier weight for his age and height.

Maybe slowing down is right for you. Ask your doctor if that's what you should be doing and for how long.

Stopping. Like slowing down, stopping asks teenagers to put the brakes on gaining weight. But stopping requires pushing harder on the brake pedal so that the gaining stops completely, for a time. Your doctor will tell you for how long to stop.

Slowing down and stopping are both wise approaches for lowering the BMI, helpful to many young people with weight problems. Yet some teenagers, especially those older and very heavy, need more. They need to lose weight. Let the doctor decide if taking off pounds is best for you; if it is, you'll likely be cautioned to lose weight slowly.

Losing weight gradually. Usually losses from a quarter pound to a pound a week are what's recommended; the BMI will decrease slowly as weight decreases gradually.

Lowering the BMI need not be a teenager's only goal. Years ago, for instance, I treated a 15-year-old boy who focused his efforts not only on reaching a healthier weight for his height but also on reducing the size of his waist. He achieved both objectives with procedures you'll soon read about which enabled him to eat better and move more. As the boy's BMI slowly decreased, so did the size of his waist—from 38 inches to 30 inches.

~~

The right goals require the right methods from the start. To be your healthiest and feel your best, talk to your doctor about what to aim for and do before you try to manage your weight.

Chapter 6
The Do's

Your goal is to lower your BMI by realistically, effectively, and healthfully managing your weight. What follows shows you how. The chapter tells you about committing yourself to and accepting responsibility for your weight management job and gives you the tools to do it. Topics include thinking upbeat thoughts, eating better, and moving more. Moreover, the chapter offers ways to make the job easier and more enjoyable.

HOW CAN I HELP MYSELF STICK TO A PROGRAM OF WEIGHT MANAGEMENT?

The short answer: COMMIT TO IT

Most of us have made promises to ourselves that we've broken later. Maybe on New Year's Eve, we've vowed to do this or that or to stop doing this or that, but 24 to 48 hours later have either forgotten the promise or decided it was just too hard to keep. And some of us wouldn't care that the commitment lasted but only a moment. Yet others of us would care so much that we would beat ourselves up for not having stuck to it, certain the failure was just more proof of being weak. But a better reason for not following through, one that doesn't assassinate character, might simply be not fully understanding what the commitment required.

Understanding your commitment is a focus of this chapter. Because lasting commitment underlies and buttresses effective weight management, this commitment is not to be made before grasping its potential costs and benefits for you. Think long and hard about what you want from effectively managing your weight, and what you'll do to make it happen. As well, be sure you agree that the buck stops with you.

About that buck, accepting it stops with you means accepting responsibility for what happens. That's what Harry S. Truman, 33rd president of the United States, would have said the words express. He kept a little sign on his desk that read, *The Buck Stops Here,* and for Truman they were words to live by. He was convinced anyone in charge of anything important should follow them and was sure they meant if something was wrong it was that person's responsibility — no one else's — to try to fix it.

Certainly your body, health, and weight qualify as important enough to try to fix, if fixing is needed. You're the person in charge of your weight. You're not the only one who cares about it, but you're the one who should care the most. Accepting that the buck stops with you doesn't mean you're to blame yourself for being too heavy. It does, however, mean agreeing to try to change, in a healthy way, what you can change to be a healthier weight. So it's up to you whether to buy one, two, or three chocolate bars at the convenience store, order one, two, or three desserts at the restaurant, eat one, two, or three hamburgers at the game, ask for an extra helpings at dinner, or play a sport after school.

Bottom line, committing to manage your weight is accepting the responsibility of working hard to manage it.

HOW CAN I TEST HOW STRONG MY COMMITMENT IS BEFORE I TRY TO LIVE UP TO IT?

Short answer: LIST COSTS, BENEFITS, BEHAVIORS, AND SPOILERS

What do you hope will happen if you live up to your weight management commitment? Here are a few possible benefits; check off those you like:

56

MY HOPE LIST:

- parents will stop nagging me about my weight
- weigh what I should for my age and sex
- become stronger
- look better on beach
- be healthier
- weigh what I should when an adult
- be able to exercise longer without tiring
- look and feel better in my clothes
- have more clothes to choose from
- stop the weight jokes at school
- stop the weight jokes at home
- date more
- do something just for me
- be invited to more parties
- feel more like I'm the boss of my body
- become more physically fit
-

List any other reasonable hopes you have, results you'd like to see.

What are you willing to do to make those hopes come true? Find out by answering the following questions; circle the *yeses*.

WHAT I WOULD DO TO MANAGE MY WEIGHT

- Are you willing to try hard to choose healthier foods, if necessary? YES NO

- Are you willing to try hard to get a family member to explore Choosemyplate with you, if necessary? (The Choosemyplate website for choosing nutritious foods and making meal plans will be described in more detail later.) YES NO

- Are you willing to try hard to not go to fast food restaurants as often, if necessary? YES NO

- Are you willing to try hard to reduce **the size and number** of your after-school snacks, if necessary? YES NO

- Are you willing to try hard to reduce **the size and number** of the helpings you usually take at lunch or at dinner, if necessary? YES NO

- Are you willing to try hard to give up some of your computer time for more sports or other vigorous activities, if necessary? YES NO

- Are you willing to try hard to give up some of your TV-watching for more energetic kinds of activity, if necessary? YES NO

- Are you willing to try hard to cut back on soft drinks, if necessary? YES NO

- Are you willing to try hard to avoid food and drink vending machines, if necessary? YES NO

- Are you willing to try hard to make healthier food and drink choices at the school cafeteria and at home, if necessary? YES NO

- Are you willing to try hard to cut down on candy, cookies, pie, and ice cream, if necessary? YES NO

- Are you willing to try hard to walk more often instead of driving or asking for rides, if necessary? YES NO

- Are you willing to try hard to track your BMI changes monthly or bimonthly? YES NO

- Are you willing to try hard to avoid the weight control snakes (to be described)?YES NO

- Are you willing to try hard to arrange opportunities for family or friends to swim, bike, walk, or run with you? YES NO

- Are you willing to try hard to enlist others to help you manage your weight? YES NO

To evaluate your commitment's strength, divide a piece of paper lengthwise, one column for *yeses* and the other for *nos*, and then total each column. More yeses means stronger resolve.

But be careful of *spoilers*. These are persuasive and usually personal reasons not to manage weight right now. To uncover those of them that might affect you, fold another piece of paper in half lengthwise, and in one column list why you should accept the weight management challenge; select reasons from your list of hopes (potential benefits). In the other column, list why you should reject the challenge (costs); reasons against managing your weight now might involve several of the weight management behaviors just mentioned.

REASONS FOR MANAGING:	REASONS FOR NOT MANAGING
- invited to more parties	- love fast food restaurants
- weight-teasing will stop	- caving in to thin-crazy world
- hate walking outside	- hate asking others for help
-clothes fit better	- embarrassing if others call attention to my having been overweight
-healthier	
-parents stop nagging about weight	
-look better on beach	
-more clothes to choose from	
-doing something just for me	
-more dates	

Now compare columns. Even though the reasons **for** managing weight outnumber those **for not** doing so, you still may doubt whether committing yourself to managing your weight right now is worth it. Some reasons against may be more important to you than all those that say go ahead, combined. Don't dismiss these *spoilers*. Even one argument against doing something now might be enough to demolish your motivation to stay committed. So, once you spot potential a *spoiler*, think about how to minimize its possible impact.

~~

Living up to a weight management commitment isn't easy. Doing so requires determination, discipline, and motivation. Doing so also requires *know how*, something the next few chapters aim to provide. In them, you'll learn practical and healthy "how-to-do- it" tips including how to eat smarter, move more, and think upbeat thoughts to enable yourself to feel good and proud of whom you are. Not every teenage weight manager will find all the advice in these what-to-do chapters pertinent and useful. But most will view much of what's said as helpful. Pick and choose from among the tips given to design a plan-of-action that fits with your needs and lifestyle. That is, construct a plan tailored to you; tailored treatments work the best.

Chapter 7
Eating Smarter

Eating is one of the great pleasures and necessities of living. Done well, it serves you well. The advice in this chapter focuses on that daily experience and how eating smarter can help you manage your weight better. Topics and tips include uncovering your eating *hotspots*, choosing the best foods, snacking better, retraining your brain, and more.

Hotspots

Tip #1 Shine a Light on Your Eating.

Tip #1, your personal detective, advises you to look closely at your eating. Search for and uncover the repeated practices, routines, and feelings that interfere with weight management (hotspots). Look for hotspots involving what, how much, where, why, and when you eat. Maybe a hotspot for you is taking too many helpings of dessert. Maybe it's taking too many helpings of dinner. Maybe it's ordering helpings that are too large when at restaurants. Maybe it's storing food in your room. Maybe it's buying food from vending machines or eating at Fast-food restaurants too often. Maybe it's what you snack on or how often you snack. Your eating has many parts and so has many potential hotspots.

Shine a light on them with the following test for uncovering eating hotspots. Think about each statement. Does it apply to you? Is it true for you? If so, put a check mark beside it, but if unsure ask parents, siblings, or friends whether they think it applies to you. Each statement highlights a potential eating hotspot.

- Having one to five regular (sugary) soft drinks a day.

- Snacking before bed.

- Taking seconds of dinner.

- Taking three or more helpings of dinner.

- Usually eating when with friends.

- Eating all the food on your plate even when no longer hungry.

- Unhappy with less than large servings when served favorite foods.

- Often eating when not hungry.

- Skipping breakfast once or more a week on average.

- Frequently gobbling down food.

- Eating or wanting to eat when seeing others eat.

- Eating or wanting to eat when or after watching food commercials on television.

- Often asking for or buying foods advertised on TV.

- Keeping food in bedroom.

- Snacking on candy or chips or similar foods when watching television or when online.

- Eating when it's time to eat even if not hungry.

- Never visiting the Choosemyplate website.

- Frequently eating at the school cafeteria.

- Going to fast food restaurants four or more times a month.

- Often buying food and drinks from vending machines.

- Frequently eating foods like candy, cookies, pie, or chips at the insistence of grandparents (or uncles, aunts, cousins, friends).

- Wanting favorite foods after seeing them, although not hungry.

- Having fewer than four *nutritional bargains* daily (foods like vegetables and fruits).

- Having more than two snacks daily.

- Ordering only the large-sizes at fast-food restaurants.

- Frequently being told to eat everything served.

- Frequently having pie, cake, cookies, or ice cream for dessert.

- Having seconds or thirds of dessert twice or more a week.

Deciding which statements apply to you is a good way to light up your eating hotspots. Another, is to observe your eating for two weeks or so. Keep a written record of your daily breakfasts, lunches, dinners, and snacks. What do you have? With whom do you eat? Eat by yourself? Are you watching TV when you eat? Where do you get your foods—vending machines, school cafeteria, fast food restaurants, home—and for which meals? Are there candy dishes in many rooms at home?

Carefully kept records that answer such questions will uncover the possibly troublesome areas of your eating. Locate them by either directly observing your eating or by taking the eating hotspot test or by doing both. Once you have a good idea of where these difficulties are, you'll know better which of the following eating smarter tips are right for you.

Choosing Foods & Meals
Smart eating is eating the right amount of the best foods every day. Smart eating is the cornerstone of healthy weight management not only for children, and adults, but also for teenagers. But how do you eat smart, if you're a teenager who's

supposed to put the brakes on gaining weight or to shed a few pounds?

Simple, say many popular magazines, some TV commercials, and a few self-proclaimed nutrition wise men: just don't eat carbs or just don't eat fats, or just down humongous amounts of grapefruit, carrots, and cauliflower every day.

Bad advice for growing teenagers. Don't listen to it. It's designed to line the pockets of its promoters at the expense of its followers. It will at best disappoint and at worst injure you. To remain healthy and strong and to grow as you should, eat the right amounts of carbohydrates, fats, and proteins daily—the three *macronutrients* required—from the highest quality foods; eat a balanced diet. Dietitians (food experts) can tell you what to eat and so can scholarly nutrition books. But there is a quicker, easier way to get that kind of information.

Tip #2 Explore Choosemyplate. Visit the Choosemyplate food guidance system at www.choosemyplate.gov. This superb one-stop shop for smarter eating tells you to:

1. *Choose healthy foods you like.*

2. *Be active every day.*

3. *Take small steps when trying to eat smarter.*

4. *Be moderate. Stay away from too many sugary and fatty foods.*

5. *Select foods from the following food groups daily:*

> (a) *Grains.* Cereals, bread, spaghetti (pasta), tortillas, and more. Grains either are whole or refined, but the whole-grains, like those in whole wheat bread, are better for you. Refined grains are those ground into smooth flour to make, for example, white bread. The refining, however, causes the grains to lose some of their nutrients, which food

manufacturers can restore. When they do they label the refined-grain product, *enriched*.

(b) *Vegetables*.

dark green vegetables like broccoli, dark green leafy lettuce, bok choy, and spinach

orange vegetables like as carrots, pumpkin, sweet potatoes, and squash

dry beans and peas (also in the protein group below) like black beans, soybeans, split peas, kidney beans, lima beans, chickpeas, navy beans, black-eyed peas, and tofu

starchy vegetables like potatoes, corn, green lima beans, and green peas

other vegetables like asparagus, Brussel sprouts, artichokes, beets, celery, cucumbers, zucchini, onions, cabbage, and green and red peppers.

(c)*Fruits*. Bananas, apples, apricots, strawberries, raspberries, cherries, lemons, limes, grapes, grapefruit, watermelon, cantaloupe, pineapple, plums, prunes, oranges, tangerines, and raisins name only some.

(d) *Milk*. Milk products include milk, yogurt, ice milk, ice cream, and cheese; all are calcium-rich to strengthen bones. When possible, choose the low in fat or fat-free milk products.

(e) *The protein group*. Beef, veal, pork, turkey, chicken, fish, eggs, nuts, seeds, beans, and peas comprise this group. Choose the fish, nuts, and seeds because they contain the kinds of oils that are good for you.

The Choosemyplate website is informative, rich with links, and from beginning to end, easy to use. In it you'll discover not only a truckload of nutritional wisdom and time-saving meal plans, but also clever tools like *MyFoodapedia* for learning about and comparing foods. As well, in it you'll read about such eating- healthier ideas as replacing refined grains with whole ones and increasing fruit in the diet.

Go to Choosemyplate, and explore it. It will help you become a smart eater and stay one, too.

Tip #3 Interact with Choosemyplate.

Click on "Choosemyplate Plan" while on the website to get to a screen for telling Choosemyplate your age, sex, and typical activities each day. After doing so, click the *submit* button, and from what you've told it, Choosemyplate will tell you the amount of grains, vegetables, fruits, milk, meat and beans, and calories you need each day.

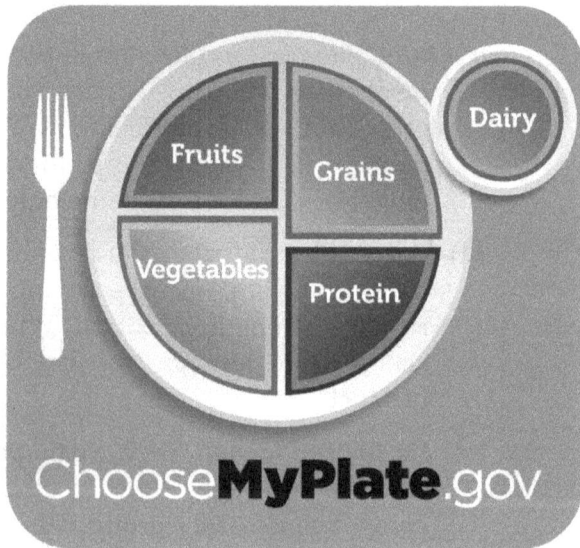

Here are a few more tips for choosing foods and meals:

Tip #4 Eat Breakfast, Lunch, and Dinner Each Day.

Tip #5 Go to Fast-Food Restaurants Less Often.

Tip #6 Plan What You'll Order Before Going to a Fast Food Restaurant.

Tip #7 Baked and Broiled Foods Are Better for You than Fried Foods.

Tip #8 For Dessert Sometimes Substitute Fresh Fruit for Pie, Cake, Cookies, and Ice Cream.

Tip #9 Drink Water More Often & Sugary Soft Drinks Less Often.

Tip #10 Eat More Vegetables and Salad At Dinner.

Snacking Smarter

Tip #11 Trick Some of Your Snack Attacks If one of your eating hotspots is snacking too often, then sometimes do something fun other than snacking. For instance, the next time you get an *I've-got-to-eat-now* urge after just having had your last planned snack of the day, try:

- playing a board game with a family member
- sending an e-mail to a friend
- writing in your diary
- listening to a CD or watching a DVD
- reading in your favorite book
- starting, continuing, or finishing a story you've authored
- drawing a picture
- playing a board game with a family member or friend

- playing badminton, riding a bike, or doing something equally as active

- walking or playing with your dog

- completing a puzzle

- challenging a family member to a game of shooting hoops indoors with a sponge ball

- challenging a family member or nearby friend to game of one-on-one basketball outside

- hitting tennis balls outside against a wall

Develop a list of favorite substitutes for snacking. And keep it handy, so you'll be ready to trick your next unwanted snack-attack.

Here are some additional smarter-snacking tips:

Tip #12 Have the Right Number of Nutritious Snacks Daily (for many teenagers that would be two).

Tip #13 Ask Your Parents to Keep Less Candy and Fewer Salty High-in-Fat Snack-foods, like Potato Chips, at Home.

Tip #14 Ask Your Parents to Keep Many Fruits and Cut Vegetables on Hand for Snacks.

Tip #15 Have More Fruit, Raw Vegetables or Cereal When Snacking Instead of Candy, Cookies, and Chips.

Tip #16 Make Snacks More Chewy by Adding Vegetables or Fruit To Them So They Last Longer.

Tip #17 Have a Special Place to Snack At Home.

Tip #18 Keep Your Own Snacks in Your Own (with your name on it) Snack Box At Home.

Tip #19 Remove Food from Your Bedroom; too Easy To Snack There

Tip #20 Remove Food from Your School Locker.

Tip #21 Ask Your Parents to Remove The Candy Dishes Near the TV & Computer.

Tip #22 Snack Less or Not At All While Watching Television or At the Computer.

Tip #23 Don't Snack (& Fill-up) On Bread While Waiting For Dinner When At Restaurants.

Tip #24 Don't Buy Snack Foods and Soft Drinks from Vending Machines.

Tip #25 Ask Friends, Grandparents, Aunts, and Uncles Not to Offer You So Many Candies, Chips, Cookies, Cakes, and Foods Like Them To Snack On.

Retraining Your Brain to Eat less

Sarah Leibovitz has big blue eyes, blonde hair, and a temper. She's just three. But she knows what she wants when it comes to rich and gooey desserts. She wants *too much*. Evidently, once after she had helped herself to a rich dessert, her parents had complained, "Sarah, that's too much." Now, *too much* and only *too much* is what she demands. "I want too much," she says when asked how much dessert to put on her plate. And either you pile it on, or she'll drown you in an ocean of tears.

Sarah's brain tells her that unless there's too much, there's too little. Her eyes have to be pleased before she'll ever permit her stomach to be pleased. Sarah's eyes, as the saying goes, are bigger than her stomach, and as a result, she's on her way to becoming a *supersizer*.

Matthew Sperling is already a supersizer. Two hours after returning home from school this robust 17-year-old sits himself down to dinner, famished. Though he'd rather play computer games than do anything else—Matt's inactive— he eats as if he regularly ran marathons and played football; in fact, jokes his family, Matt's appetite rivals Godzilla's. Soon, Matt's dad fills

71

the boy's dinner plate with salad and corn and with what Matt loves and voraciously devours: a quarter pound grilled to perfection hamburger patty. Gone in 40 seconds. Matt feels cheated, wants more burger, much more burger.

Choosemyplate tells us how much food from each food group we require each day. Seventeen year-old inactive Matt, for instance, needs 6 ½oz from the protein group, which would include the hamburger he wolfed down at dinner, the tuna he had at lunch, and the peanut butter he enjoyed at breakfast. Six and one half ounces of such foods is, Choosemyplate says, enough for him from this group for one day. Would you consider it enough for you?

Many of today's teenagers would not for themselves. They'd feel that 6 ½oz in a day is way too little, especially if they routinely frequent drive-throughs for pound-sized hamburgers, double size containers of french fries, and 16 ounce colas. And too little, especially if they prefer the restaurants that serve massive steaks, Caesar salads, and butter-slathered baked potatoes. And too little, especially if they live in families who regularly offer only the largest of meat meals along with the richest of desserts. Indeed, supersized amounts of meat and other foods is the reality for numbers of today's adolescents, many of whom grow overweight or obese. Not all supersizers will become too heavy, but those who do and continue to supersize will remain so.

Are your eyes bigger than your stomach? Do food portions have to be enormous for you even to think you'll be, let alone actually be, satisfied? If so, your brain is telling you to supersize to be content. Therefore, to stop supersizing, you'll have to retrain your brain.

*Tip #26 Retrain Your Brain To Take Smaller Portions at Home &
Restaurants.* You can do that at home by *gradually* cutting down on how much food you take with each helping, and similarly you can do that at restaurants by cutting down the size of your

food and drink orders. After a while, your eyes won't need to see so much food before you're pleased, and your stomach won't need to contain so much before you're full; choosing smaller portions will have become acceptable and comfortable.

Tip #27 Retrain Your Brain To Take Fewer Helpings. Retrain your brain to be satisfied with not only smaller portions but also fewer helpings. Talk to your parents about what you want to do and why. Be sure to let them know you aren't trying some crackpot diet. You just want to cut back on the number of helpings you take at dinner and at other meals.

When retraining your brain so you can eat less:

- Don't obsess over the size of portions and number of servings; pay attention to how much you're eating, but don't feel compelled to count calories.

- Don't try to change everything all at once; the gradual approach works far better.

- Don't undercut Choosemyplate guidelines, unless a doctor or dietitian, directs you to; reduce portions and servings sensibly and healthfully.

- Don't complicate your task unnecessarily; look for simple ways to reduce portions and servings, such as:

    choosing smaller sizes at fast food restaurants

    having fresh fruit instead of more helpings of the Main dish

    adding vegetables to some snacks to make them more nutritious and chewy

    eating slower so that smaller portions last longer and are more filling.

Tip #28 Retrain Your Brain To Eat When Hungry, Stop When Full.

Young children do this quite well, yet their parents are often unhappy when they do. But parents should be glad instead because it's more natural and far better that hunger rather than the sight of food compel a child to eat; the same reasoning applies to adults and teenagers.

Don't eat just because there's food on your plate or just because you see and smell good food or, as the following story from my doctor-friend illustrates, just because you notice the hour is late:

"It was hot enough to fry eggs on the sidewalk my second day in Las Vegas, and to bronze my pasty-white body, I was sunbathing by the resort's luxurious pool. While dozing there, I was jolted awake by this piercing shout, actually more of a wail. I thought somebody was having a heart attack, but that wasn't it at all. A nearby fellow sunbather, about 70 pounds overweight who sounded as if he'd just remembered that he'd forgotten to turn off his stove 2000 miles to the east, was panicking. The reason he was upset, however, was I later learned, strapped to his wrist. Evidently, he'd looked at his watch and, realizing it was 10 minutes past noon, had panicked. He was, he thought, missing out on lunch. So feeling desperate, he had bolted from his pool-chair and headed for the line of guests waiting for the noon buffet. This feast was just one of five the resort offered throughout the day, every day, for free; actually, they were included in the price of the room."

Most likely, hunger had less to do with igniting this man's passion for food than did his suddenly realizing his time to eat was ticking away. The man had either lost, misplaced, or rejected his inborn hunger-eating connection.

Have you lost, misplaced, or rejected yours? If so, try to regain it. Having it back will loosen the outside world's stranglehold on your eating, and as a result, you'll probably eat less overall. Having it back will also free you from the calculated tugs on your appetite crafted by fancy-food displays advertised on TV, in magazines, and on billboards. The advertisers won't be happy, but you'll be.

Here are a few more tips on when to begin and end meals:

Tip #29 Let Moderate, Not Intense, Hunger Guide You. Don't allow yourself to become so deprived of food that when it arrives your control vanishes.

Tip #30 Don't Purposely Starve During the Day in Order to Stuff at Night. The starving-stuffing routine contradicts the healthy approach to weight management.

Tip #31 Don't Eat Just Because The Foods You See On TV Plead, "Try Me You'll Love Me." Eat Because You're Hungry.

Tip #32 Don't Eat Just Because Others Are Eating. Eat Because You're Hungry.

Tip #33 Eat Slower and Chew More Thoroughly To Feel Fuller.

Chapter 8
Moving More

The two biggest *Do's* of healthy weight management are eating better and moving more. However, far too many teens set on reaching a healthier weight zero in only on eating better. They downplay or entirely forget about such rewards of moving more as:

- a healthier weight throughout your life
- greater flexibility
- better posture
- easier time breathing after exerting yourself
- more energy
- stronger bones and muscles
- more fit
- greater endurance
- lower risk of type 2 diabetes
- lower risk of some cancers
- lower risk of heart disease
- greater self-esteem
- increased alertness
- greater sense of well-being
- easier to keep trim

This chapter says to remember and not minimize the rewards of moving more and offers advice (tips) on how to become and stay active.

Activating

You do many activities every day. Some, like watching television and playing checkers, chess, or computer games are done sitting down. Others, like tennis, jogging, running, gymnastics, basketball, biking, swimming, weight lifting, martial arts, football, baseball, hiking, biking, dancing, and walking, require moving. Both kinds can be fun but only the moving-more type help manage weight.

And only the moving- more type, like swimming, walking a mile at a good pace, and jogging slowly, speed up heart rate, improve breathing, and cause sweating from exertion. Such activities can be done for extended periods without gasping for air while doing them or collapsing on the ground when finishing. More grueling and fast-paced activities, however (for example, volleyball, swimming laps, running, sprinting, tennis, and racquetball), will cause breathlessness, but get easier with practice. No matter which moving more activities become a part of your life, they'll all help you manage your weight if they help you become active long enough each day. But what's long enough?

Tip #34 Get At Least Sixty Minutes of Moving-more Activity Each Day. Every day. Work up to the hour slowly, and remember you need not do it all at once. If you prefer, break it up into shorter bursts, maybe 15 to 20 minutes of activity at a time throughout the day. And don't count routines like bathing, walking from one room to the other at home, emptying garbage, washing clothes, or ironing pants, and so forth as part of the activity hour; they're important, of course, so by all means continue to do them, but just don't figure them into your total activity time. Also, realize 60 minutes of activity a day is a MINIMUM; doing more is more than okay.

Tip #35 Discover Your Activity-likes. From all the sports and active games there are, make a list of those you *know* you like.

That's your *activity-like* list. Then, write down all those activities you *might* like and find out which of them could become actual *activity-likes*. One way to do that is:

Select a few of the might-likes to try. Using the chart below, list your choices in the ACTIVITIES I HOPE TO DO column. Do as many of them as possible. Record those you actually did in the ACTIVITIES I DID column of the chart. Rate each of those you did in column three. Use the 4-choice rating scheme below.

MY ACTIVITIES CHART   DAY & DATE:

ACTIVITIES I HOPE TO DO	ACTIVITIES I DID	RATING

ACTIVITY RATING: Copy as many charts as you need
1= HATED IT   2= DISLIKED IT
3= OKAY   4= LIKED IT

After three weeks of charting, you'll know more about your *activity-likes* and may find some new enjoyable ways to move more.

Another way to discover fun activities is to visit the BAM (BODY AND MIND) web site at www.bam.gov/index.html and click on the physical activity link. This will take you to the activity- suggestion page and a quiz. The quiz asks what's most important to you about an activity: doing it with friends, being challenged by it, having it be fast-paced, and more. Once BAM has this kind of information, it can and will suggest activities that fit you best.

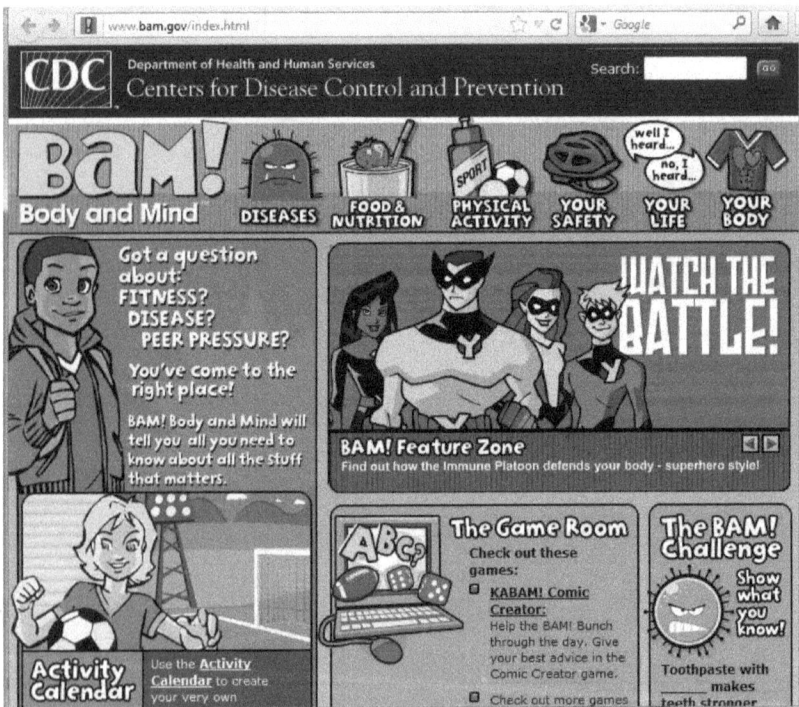

Planning Activities &Getting Yourself To Do Them

Tip #36 Make A Weekly Activity Plan. Here's how:

1) From your list of *activity-likes,* choose some you intend to do.

2) Write down when and where and about how long and with whom you'll do them.

3) Identify what you need to do them (for instance, bike or tennis racket and ball).

4) Make sure you can easily get this equipment— perhaps you already own it or know someone else who does.

Now, after having planned what to do, encourage yourself to live up to your plan. Easier said than done. Becoming more of a mover is hard, especially when you're quite comfortable with the sit-down life. If motivating yourself to get off the couch or away from the TV and computer screens even for a little while seems harder than earning a scholarship to Harvard, ask your parents for help. The next tip describes what they can do.

Tip#37 Pay for Progress. The pay for progress method motivates you to move more by rewarding you in two ways for moving. First, there is *Pay* for becoming more active. The pay (money, prizes, or points towards the money and prizes) you receive soon after achieving a moving-more goal. The pay is like earning a salary for doing a job well. It's not a bribe any more than is the money you're paid for the work you do or the grade you get for the scholarship you show. It's not blackmail either, if it stops you from staying at an unhealthy weight. The pay just boosts motivation; it just nudges you towards becoming more active.

The second way you're rewarded is by experiencing the benefits of more moving, like feeling better and lowering your BMI. Seeing such progress lifts spirits, boosts motivation, and elevates self-esteem.

To try out the pay for progress method in order to build a daily hour of activity, follow these steps:

MAKE A DEAL WITH YOUR PARENTS. Tell them you want to work up to doing 60 minutes of vigorous activity each day, but need help motivating yourself. Ask them if they'll pay you a designated amount, from $.10 up to $.50 for every minute up to 60 minutes you play sports or do something as vigorous. [All told, that's somewhere between $6 and $30 dollars for an hour of activity.] Also, tell them that you'll progress gradually towards the 60 minute, record how you'll reach it, and only after reaching it, ask to be paid the agreed upon amount.

EARN YOUR FIRST 10 REWARD POINTS. Be active for 10 minutes. Maybe walk, run, swim, or ride a bike for 10 minutes. Then, give yourself 10 points. Each of these points represents one minute of being active and is worth whatever you have agreed a minute of activity is worth—somewhere between a dime and 50 cents.

EARN YOUR SECOND 10 REWARD POINTS. Now, be active for 20 minutes, and upon reaching the 20 minute mark, give yourself another 10 points.

EARN YOUR THIRD 10 REWARD POINTS. When active for 30 minutes, give yourself 10 more points. So the idea is to add 10 points of earnings for each 10 minute increase of activity until attaining the 60 minute goal. Getting there may take days or weeks, but getting there you will.

RECORD EARNINGS. Keep track of points on a computer, in a diary, or on a chart in your bedroom. Watch your earnings grow to experience the very rewarding sign of becoming more active.

CASH IN POINTS. When you have 60 points, cash them in for the amount of money agreed to.

Here's an even simpler way to apply the pay for progress method.

Let's say you're a 15-year-old boy named Danny. You spend much of your time either at school or in front of the TV or playing video games or petting Wilson the family's seven-year-old golden retriever. Your BMI is 24.2, so you're overweight.

Deciding to start doing something about your weight, you propose this deal to your parents: "If I walk Wilson 30 minutes daily for three months, will you pay me enough to spend a day with Mike and Pat at Fun Mountain amusement park or at the Crenshaw Waterslide?" They say yes, and after some discussion agree to award you 10 points for each 30 minute dog-walk. You keep track of the minutes and points. After earning 200 reward points, you can cash them in for the admission price of one outing.

It's agreed that the deal is to last three months and that you can have as many outings as earned. Three months go by, and you have enjoyed going to Fun Mountain twice. Everyone is happy with the way the deal has worked and so decide to try it again. Three more months go by (it's six months later) and you've not only been to Fun Mountain several times, but also to the Crenshaw waterslide twice. What's more, to everyone's delight, your BMI is now nearly out of the overweight range.

Pay for progress deals work best when they reward behaviors such as playing more sports or snacking less on cookies. Also they work best when they're written and clear about what the rewards are and how to earn them. Pay for progress deals can be simple like Danny's or more elaborate like the one you'll read about later for Terri Melendez. They also can be used to help you eat smarter, think better (discussed later), and talk assertively (discussed earlier).

Staying Active

Tip#38 Make Being Active Fun. Enjoy being activity to keep being active. One way to make any activity more fun is to do it with others. So maybe invite your father to swim with you or ask your mom or a friend from school to bike with you. Or possibly challenge your brother or sister to a game of badminton or tennis. The possibilities are numerous.

Two more tips on staying active:

Tip#39 Be Active in Many Ways, But Don't Overdo It.

Tip# 40 Make Rainy Day Activity Plans. Don't Let Bad Weather Idle You.

Chapter 9
Feeling Better: Thinking Upbeat Thoughts & Talking Back to Yourself

Part of chapter 1 focused on the importance of standing up for your rights and how being assertive can help do that. The message was: when possible, talk back to others who bring you down. The message here at least as important is talk back to yourself, if it is you attacking your self-esteem. This is because what you say to yourself (that is think) determines how you'll feel and ultimately what you'll do. So, with regard to taking charge of your weight, if you think constructively, you'll be more likely to act constructively.

Conversely, think destructively, you'll be more likely to act destructively. Telling yourself, *I'll quit without really trying, I'm just too weak to stick this out* increases the chances of quitting prematurely. Telling yourself, I don't have what it takes to do anything about my weight reduces the chances of doing something about your weight long enough and well enough to get the desired results.

Likewise, you make the mission harder and more stressful by telling yourself:

- either I'll follow all my plans to eat better, or I'll quit this planning.

- either I'll have washboard abs in six months, or I'll stop exercising completely.

- either I'll totally succeed in managing my weight, or I'll be forever unhappy.

Such thinking, as mentioned, is **all-or-nothing** thinking. To all or nothing thinkers, either something is good or bad, perfect or flawed, beautiful or ugly, successful or failing. With the all-or-

85

nothing thought, the only possibility after the "all" is the "nothing." There's no pretty good, no less than perfect, no just kind of cute, no somewhat successful — no shades of gray between the extremes, no wiggle room. All or nothing thinking demands too much from teenage weight managers and tolerates too little from them. No setbacks permitted. But the road to a healthier weight is rarely smooth. Setbacks happen. And when they do, rigid all or nothing thinkers will feel defeated, weak, incompetent, sometimes unworthy, and frequently hopeless. And then in despair, adding injury to insult, they'll likely quit their journey to a healthier weight.

As derailing as all or nothing thinking, perhaps even more derailing, is the steady barrage of never-ending, paralysing, and demeaning anti-fat propaganda heavy teenagers face daily. It can generate strong feelings of despair and futility that disrupt their continuing struggle to reach a healthier weight.

As said earlier, many people of all ages and occupations (including numbers of healthcare professionals) assume and freely proclaim that the heavy lack the willpower, beauty, and ability of those who aren't heavy. One of my most influential and unforgettable teachers, my eighth-grade physical education and math teacher, was just such a person.

The man, Mr. L., clearly despised heaviness. Mr. L. was himself what you'd call a V-shape — broad shoulders, small waist — who delighted in wearing his shirt two buttons open at the top as he strutted about the classroom and playing fields. He was convinced that boys who weren't muscular or thin, couldn't be very good at much of anything, particularly sports, and so couldn't be one of his chosen few. True, he never actually said that but his actions, like buying treats for only thin and muscular athletic kids and snubbing fat ones, clearly and unmistakably conveyed it. Mr. L. was sure which boys were and were not worthy, and because to most guys he was the person to emulate, most of us agreed with him. We unhesitatingly adopted his

86

view: *if you're heavy, you must be weak; if you're heavy, you'll never be good at sports; if you're heavy, you must be unpopular.*

Those heavy teens and preteens who believe such nonsense (I confess I did years ago) are on a slippery slope to despair and depression. They are likely to hold one or more of the following 20 demeaning and self-disparaging assumptions/thoughts:

BRINGING-MYSELF-DOWN ASSUMPTIONS/ THOUGHTS

1. If I'm too heavy, I'm ugly.

2. If I'm too heavy, others won't like me.

3. If I'm too heavy, I must change fast, NO MATTER HOW.

4. If I'm too heavy, I won't have any friends.

5. If I'm too heavy, there's nothing I can do about it.

6. If I stay too heavy, I'll always be alone.

7. If I'm too heavy, I can't be happy.

8. If I'm too heavy, I should be ashamed.

9. If I'm too heavy, I can't let others see me exercise.

10. If I'm too heavy, I'm not as good as those who aren't.

11. If I'm too heavy, I can't be popular.

12. If I'm too heavy, I hate my body.

13. If I'm too heavy, I'll always be teased or bullied.

14. If I'm too heavy, I deserve to be teased and made fun of.

15. If I'm too heavy, I have little self-control and not enough willpower.

16. If I'm too heavy, I must be lazy.

17. If I'm too heavy, I'm unworthy.

18. If I'm too heavy, I hate everything about me.

19. If I'm too heavy, I should hide.

20. If I'm too heavy, that's who I am... all that I am.

Be wary of these self esteem-thieves. One or more of them could rule your mood without your even knowing. You might know only that when something unpleasant reminds you that you're heavy, you feel so sad or angry and so hopeless and desperate that you consider taking diet pills, fasting, purposely vomiting after eating, or something as harmful and nonsensical. These actions are the snakes of weight mismanagement; we'll say more about such vipers later.

Don't become their prey. If ever you feel so bad about your weight that you might succumb to one of them, seek help. Talk to the school's guidance counselor, your parents, your doctor. As well, try what the next tip suggests.

Tip#41 Talk back to Those Who Bring You Down: Others & Yourself.

Chapter 2 discussed how to, when to, and when not to talk back to others bullying you for being heavy. Talking back to yourself for bullying yourself with self- disparaging thoughts is procedurally somewhat different, as you'll now see:

- First, identify what it is you're thinking that bothers you. Ask yourself: *What am I telling myself right now* or *What thoughts are going through my mind right now.* Second, talk back to each of these thoughts by questioning how true, how fair, or how sensible it is. You might ask questions like:

- How do I know that what I'm telling myself is really true — what's the evidence?

- Is what I'm telling myself really fair to me?

• Would I tell another kid like me to think that way about himself or herself? If not why would I be kinder to him or her than to me?

When asking such questions, step outside of yourself to answer. Pretend you're somebody else talking to you; the other person wants to know the truth and fairness of what you're telling yourself.

For example, let's say for the past three days you've been trying to eat better to manage your weight. Tonight, two hours after dinner, you feel like snacking and decide on having an orange — good choice. Fresh fruit is in the refrigerator. You open the refrigerator door intent on having the fruit, but see a huge slice of cherry pie first. Irresistible, so you enjoy the pie. Upon finishing, however, you're unreasonably upset — quite angry at yourself and sad at the same time.

Step 1. Identify your thoughts. *What are you thinking or assuming and then telling yourself?* Your answer might be:

1) How come I did that?

2) I can't say 'No' to pie or donuts or ice cream.

3) I'll always be too heavy, I can't change that.

4) I'm just too heavy and ugly.

But what are you really telling yourself? To answer that critical question, let's analyze the sentences one by one in terms of the 20 *bringing-myself-down* assumptions/thoughts just named. Compare each sentence with each assumption/thought on this list to see what each sentence is truly saying.

1. How come I did that? [not on the list, just a question]

2. I can't say 'No' to pie or donuts or ice cream. [This is close to #15 on the list: "If I'm too heavy, I have little self-control and not enough willpower."]

3. I'll always be too heavy, I can't change that. [This is close to #5 on the list: " If I'm too heavy, there's nothing I can do about it."]

4. I'm just too heavy and ugly.[This is #1 on the list: "If I'm too heavy, I'm ugly."]

Step 2. Talk back to the nasty thoughts the sentences express by questioning each sentence. [Use words most meaningful to you when talking back.]

1. Bringing-myself-down thought #15: "If I'm too heavy, I have little self-control and not enough willpower."Your talk-back to #15 might question the evidence that all heavy teenagers have too little self-control and your conclusion might be:

> "When they want to, many heavy teenagers can show that they have control over what they eat. So just because you're heavy doesn't mean you haven't self-control. There are many times I show control. Just because I had something that I later wished I hadn't in no way means I lack self-control. Sometimes I can have things like pie. Having it once in awhile doesn't mean I'm going to have it every chance I get. I still have plenty of self-control."

2. Bringing-myself-down thought #5: "If I'm too heavy, there's nothing I can do about it." Your talk-back to #5 might again question the evidence. Who says you can't do anything about it? Your conclusion might be:

> "There's no proof I can't do anything about my weight. Many other heavy teens have eventually learned to manage weight. So can I. I snacked on pie instead of an orange. No big deal. Once in awhile is okay and doesn't mean there's nothing I can do about being heavy."

90

3. *Bringing-myself-down thought #1*: "If I'm too heavy, I'm ugly."

Your talk- back to #1 should question the evidence, logic, and fairness of this thought/assumption. Your conclusion could be:

"It's unfair for me to say that. I wouldn't say that to Roberta or Robbie. They're as heavy as I am, and they're not ugly. Just because you're heavy doesn't mean you're ugly. NO MATTER HOW HEAVY I AM, OR FOR HOW LONG I'M HEAVY, I'M NOT UGLY."

If you need extra help in dealing with such negative thoughts about yourself, talk with your parents and doctor about finding a specialist in cognitive behavior therapy.

~~

Think better to feel better.

Chapter 10
Stimulus Control

I teach psychology at a local University. Several years ago, two days before the final exam in my class on abnormal psychology, a very upset student came to see me. He knocked loudly on my office door. As soon as I saw him, I knew something was wrong: his eyes were blood red, his hair looked like it hadn't been combed for a week, and his forehead was dripping with sweat.

"I want to go to Psychology graduate school and get a Masters degree. I need a good grade in your class to get in, and I know I can do better in abnormal psych than I have been," he said.

"Well, how are you doing?" He just stared at me without speaking, so I went on, "What's the problem?"

"I can't seem to study well this term. I just moved into the new University Dorm. I always fall asleep whenever I study there. All my classes are suffering."

He sounded desperate. "Tell me how you go about studying for my class," I asked.

"Three days before each of your tests, I try to cram the material into my head six hours each night after dinner. The library on campus is a zoo after six in the evening, so I stay in my dorm room. My roommate is quiet, but outside in the dorm halls it's noisy."

"How come you fall asleep when you're studying? Do you fall asleep at your desk?"

"I guess the material bores me." I squirmed a little, but wasn't really offended. "I don't like my desk; the chair's too hard, so I study in bed. Why can't I study better?"

I knew why. BAD stimulus   control because he was studying at the wrong time, in the wrong place, and in the wrong way. He was studying after dinner in bed (probably sleepy), and he was cramming— trying to learn too much in too little time. His problem was bad stimulus control of studying. To turn his bad stimulus control into good stimulus control, he needed to rearrange his world so he could study at a better time (like after dinner), in a better place (like at a desk or table), and in a better way — gradually instead of cramming.

Tip#42 Practice Good Stimulus Control of Your Eating & Activity. The following 23 rearrangements exemplify stimulus control maneuvers that will make it easier to eat smarter and move more. Try those that feel right for you.

1. Have snacking-urges initiate something enjoyable other than eating (see tip # 11).

2. Ask friends to stop pushing you to eat candies, cookies, fries, and so on.

3. Ask parents to store leftovers in non-see-through containers, so the foods are less likely to be grabbed.

4. Designate where you'll eat, and don't eat anywhere else.

5. Ask parents to keep on hand lots of vegetables and fruits.

6. Ask parents to stop telling you to clean your plate.

7. Ask parents not to keep many high-fat foods at home.

8. Ask parents not to keep many ready to eat packaged foods at home.

9. Remove from your bedroom any foods you keep there.

10. Ask to remove candy dishes from the TV room.

11. Keep your snacks, except vegetables and fruits, in your own snack-food container. Write your name on the container.

94

12 .Eat less often in front of the television and while reading or listening to music.

13. Avoid school vending machines.

14. Remove foods from your school locker.

15. Avoid as often as possible fatty cafeteria foods. Take your lunch to school.

16. Ask servers at restaurants to serve the bread with and not before the main meal.

17. Learn the menus of restaurants you frequent.

18. Plan when to exercise.

19.Plan where to exercise.

20. Plan how to exercise and what you'll do if plans have to change.

21. Have exercise apparel and equipment (e.g., bike) ready.

22. Include friends when playing sports, taking walks, going for runs, and so forth.

23. Move more, but don't stop all enjoyable sit-down games and recreations. Find time for both.

~ ~

Practicing good stimulus control will help you do the weight management job well. Practicing the tips described next will help you stay well while doing it.

Chapter 11
Sidestep the Seductive Snakes of Senseless Slimming

There's too much misinformation from too many misinformed people about the best way to control weight. Recognizing this, the previous chapters have provided informed tips on what to do to manage weight the right way— the *do's*.

This chapter provides informed tips on what not to do while attempting to manage weight the right way—the *don'ts*. Each *don't* is a weight mismanagement snake—a needless, nonsensical, disappointing, or dangerous slimming practice or side effect to avoid. Teenagers desperate for instant solutions are the most susceptible to them; the list that follows names 10 of the worst snakes.

Ten Poisonous Snakes of Weight Mismanagement

1. Seeking miracle cures to manage weight

2. Taking nonprescription diet pills to manage weight.

3. Becoming a slave to the scale when managing weight

4. Fasting or skipping meals to manage weight.

5. Purposely purging food to manage weight

6. Believing that managing weight will solve all your problems (putting too much on the line)

7. Stopping weight management efforts in the face of presumed failure (giving up on yourself)

8. Thinking what you weigh is who you are

9. Obsessing over calories

10. Making never again promises about so-called forbidden foods

Tip#43 Don't Seek "Miracle" Cures. Abracadabra and.... Magic is fun.

What teenage boy wouldn't love to be able to wave a wand and presto, have what he wants? What teenage girl wouldn't love to be able to drink a potion and presto, rid herself of what she doesn't want?

Unfortunately, however, there are no magical answers to weight problems. Still that doesn't stop some teenagers from wishing that there were.

And it doesn't stop some shady characters from claiming that there are and getting rich swearing that there are. Charlatans like them have been around for a long time. Years ago, for instance, they were the fast-talking con men who traveled from town to town selling so-called "miracle cures." These hucksters would trick the more desperate townsfolk with promises of freedom from aches and pains. But the promises were as worthless as the pricey bottles of colored water the con men lied about to sell. Such useless products eventually came to be called *snake oil.*

Snake oil salesmen (and saleswomen, too) are still alive and well. Yet they no longer need to ride into towns on wagons. Instead, they can slink into homes on TV screens or advertise their potions, powders, miracle drinks, no-strain exercise gimmicks, and "magic diets" in magazines for teenagers. These fakes still want your cash and still won't provide much in return for it. So stay away from their snake oils and effort-free workout schemes. All junk. Stay away from their "magic diets," too. The diets cost too much and give back too little, likely robbing you of many of the nutrients you need. Play it safe, and unless a doctor or dietitian says otherwise, avoid going on any special diet.

Probably, few of you think of "diet" as a road to good nutrition and health. Probably, instead, you consider it as:

- discomfort, restriction, and denial

- something to start and then stop

- something almost mystical

- something with strict rules forbidding certain foods and promoting others

Perhaps, like Garfield (cartoonist Jim Davis), you believe that "diet" is Die with a T. But a better way to think of "diet" is as the Greeks long ago defined it: a way to live — *Diaita*. Make the word "diet" mean a comfortable, lasting, and prosperous approach to eating and exercising that you can enjoy for life.

Tip#44 Don't Take Non-prescription Diet Pills. Leave them in the pharmacies and markets that sell them. Not only won't they work for you, but some work against you. Some contain harmful ingredients linked to blood pressure difficulties, heart rhythm problems, and nervous system irregularities. Over-the-counter diet pills have no place in the life of a healthy teenager

Tip#45 Don't Become A Slave to The Scale. Don't jump on a scale every chance you get to see if you've lost any weight. Maybe you're not even supposed to be dropping weight. Perhaps instead, for a specified time, the prescription is just not gaining at all. So, if reducing isn't the objective, why keep checking if you are?

Even if the doctor okays losing as your goal, don't jump on the scale every few hours or days to see if you are losing. One reason why not to is that many weight scales, especially those easy-to-trip-over types found in most home bathrooms, are untrustworthy. So often do they mislead, those teenagers who tie their moods to them may feel triumphant one day and desperate the next when in fact nothing really positive or negative has happened either time. By all means keep track of your weight,

99

just don't over check it and become a slave to scales. Monthly checks usually are good enough.

Tip#46 Don't Fast or Skip Meals. Fasting is temporarily starving. Done too often, it will make you nauseous, dizzy, constipated, and weak. What's more, it may, because fasting prevents you from eating enough carbohydrate, give you horribly foul breath (halitosis) that smells like metal and tastes like it, too. The longer the fast, the worse the side effects. Prolonged fasts can kill.

Also, for some young women in particular, fasting serves a self-destructive mind-game that begins with thinking *I must fast and keep fasting so that I keep losing* and ends with becoming a walking-talking-skeleton. The game has triggered a potentially deadly eating disorder, *anorexia nervosa*. Those trapped by *anorexia nervosa* starve themselves because they fear becoming heavy and fat, if they eat even slightly more than a parakeet would.

Unless medical or religious reasons require fasting, don't fast. Don't skip meals, either. Actually, skipping meals to control weight is just a form of inappropriate fasting that can cloud thinking and dull the senses. As well, in a strange twist of fate, skipping meals can actually cause more not less eating. Going to school with the stomach on empty and then skipping lunch, too, will leave one starving by the time school ends. As a result, the normal after-school desire to eat will likely explode into a voracious hard-to-satisfy hunger, appeasable only by nonstop snacking.

Tip#47 Don't Purge On Purpose. Purposely purging food, something bulimics do, is harmful, foolish, and ineffective — you can't purge all calories just consumed. Purging is fear-driven behavior. Those with the eating disorder of bulimia are, like anorexics, deathly afraid of becoming fat.

100

But unlike most anorexics, bulimics fuel the fear by binging before they purge. When binging, done usually alone, bulimics gobble humongous quantities of food. Favorites include cookies, crackers, candy, cakes, potato chips, french fries, ice cream, pie, sliced meat, buckets of chicken, and the like.

Whatever she chooses to binge on, the bulimic teen (most likely a young female) feels controlled by food, compelled to eat it all. Once it's gone, and she's free of the need to binge, however, she's overpowered by the urge to purge. Anxiously, desperately, she now wants to rid herself of what's just been eaten and feel empty. So she may search her purse for laxatives to swallow—one patient I know would take 50 after each binge—and nervously wait for them to force her to poop. Or more commonly, she may fast walk, even run to the nearest sink or toilet, stick two fingers or a toothbrush far down into her throat to gag, bend over, and vomit.

Scarf and barf. That's what students and teachers in some colleges, high schools, and middle schools call the binging/vomiting routine. The scarf and barf nickname implies how nasty and disgusting the practice becomes, especially to the young woman it traps.

And trapped she is. The ritual not only vice-grips her—she can't stop—but also likely compromises her health. She may become clinically depressed because of it. She may, from abusing laxatives, lose the ability to move her bowels naturally. She may, because of repeatedly vomiting, rip holes in the food tube that runs from her throat to her stomach (the esophagus) or rot the enamel that covers her teeth, ruining her smile. She may cause her heart to beat irregularly. This happens because too much vomiting drains the body of the vital potassium it needs for the heart to beat as it should.

So, even if done only occasionally, purging food to control weight is unwholesome, unhealthy, and unnecessary. It's a truly vicious snake.

Tip#48 Don't Put Too Much on the Line. Managing weight successfully can jump start feeling better in many areas. But, by itself, isn't likely to be the answer to everything that might be upsetting you. So if shy, angry, depressed, whatever your issues, talk about them with the school's guidance counselor or another trained professional.

Tip#49 Don't give up on trying to help yourself. Let's say that for the past 10 months you've been struggling to reach a better weight, but aren't any lighter. Perhaps, however, you're not supposed to be any lighter; you are older and most likely taller now, so you would expect to be heavier.

Perhaps your body mass index (BMI) is less now than when you started 10 months ago. That's progress. Then again, maybe your BMI hasn't changed over the 10 months. Does that mean you've failed? No. Success may still be yours to claim:

- perhaps you're now eating more nutritiously

- perhaps you're now taking smaller portions and fewer servings

- perhaps you're now playing sports more often

- perhaps you're now confronting classmates and relatives who tease you about your weight

- perhaps you're now talking to (thinking about) yourself more positively

Check carefully what's changed, and consult with those you trust about what to do next. Maybe they'll urge you to continue on the same path. If so, and you forge ahead, yet still can't lower your BMI after months of trying to, ask about getting special help. Your doctor or guidance counselor might recommend a behavior therapist specializing in weight management.

Whatever you do, don't give up on yourself by quitting your weight management program or endanger yourself physically by rigidly dieting, taking nonprescription diet pills, purging, and so forth.

And don't devastate yourself psychologically by doing what the next tip cautions against.

Tip#50 Don't Think What You Weigh Is Who You Are. Your weight, a physical characteristic, is just one of your many characteristics. You have an abundance of virtues, talents, and behaviors. Who you are is not, never has been, and never will be what you weigh.

Two more snakes to avoid:

Tip #51 Don't Count Calories Obsessively. Obsessive calorie counting has been described in the chapter on CONCERNS.

Tip #52 Don't Make "Never Again Promises" about So-called Forbidden Foods. This snake was also discussed earlier in the chapter on CONCERNS.

~~

Avoid all the snakes of weight mismanagement. In the long run, you'll be happier and healthier if you do.

Chapter 12
Cautions

To help you take charge of your weight everyday, this book has suggested targets to focus on and tips to consider. You've learned about:

- eating smarter (including finding your eating hotspots, visiting Choosemyplate, and snacking smarter)

- retraining your brain to downsize your food supply

- practicing good stimulus control to rearrange your food world

- moving more

- thinking upbeat thoughts

- talking back assertively to anyone attempting to bring you down, which includes yourself

- avoiding the snakes of weight mismanagement.

Now, it's important for you to scrutinize the 20 cautions listed next; many are the *don'ts* we've called snakes.

CAUTIONS TO BE MINDFUL OF BEFORE AND WHILE MANAGING YOUR WEIGHT

1) Talk with Your Parents about Your Intentions

2) Talk with the Family Doctor about Your Intentions

3) Accept Responsibility for Managing Your Weight

4) Commit to Trying Hard to Manage Your Weight

5) Seek Support from Others like Parents & Friends

6) Realize that Managing Your Weight Doesn't Require Giving-up TV, Computer Time, and All Other Sit-down Activities

7) Ask Your Doctor If You Should or Shouldn't Try to Lose Weight

8) Be Patient and Gradual When Making Changes

The eighth caution is particularly important when it comes to losing weight. If reducing is what's best for you, the doctor may counsel you to lose no more than a quarter pound to a pound a week. Resist the temptation to speed up that pace because taking off too much too quickly is unhealthy for a growing teenager. The feeling *I'll do anything to lose weight fast* could push you into the snake pit of dangerous weight loss schemes.

9) Seek Nutritious Foods & Nutritional Bargains

10) Don't Obsess over Calories

11) If You Do Have to Lose Weight, Don't Become a Slave to Scales

12) Don't Seek Miracle Cures: Snake Oil, No-strain Fixes, or Magic Diets

13) Don't Fast or skip meals

14) Don't Purposely Purge Food

15) Don't Take Nonprescription Diet Pills

16) Don't Diet, Unless a Doctor or Dietitian Says To

17) Don't Make "Never-again Promises" about so-called "Forbidden Foods"

18) Don't Give-up Trying When Results Aren't What You Want

19) Don't Think Managing Your Weight Is the Answer to All Your Problems

20) Don't Think How Heavy You Are Is Who You Are

Chapter 13
The Case of Terri Melendez

Fourteen -year-old Terresa Melendez (Terri for short) had had enough of Maggie McKenzie & Lujane Heart, two girls in her grade 9 algebra class at Viscount Alexander. Even though the three had been good friends up until grade 6, Maggie and Lujane had been continually and regularly ridiculing Terri about her weight. At the start of grade 8, Terri weighed 115 pounds but by the end of the school year and over the summer had put on 20 pounds. So, by grade 9, 5 feet tall Terri was 135 pounds. Her body mass index at that time was 26.4, larger than that of 93% of the other girls her age. Terri, therefore, was decidedly overweight.

Terri hated being teased, sometimes so much so she didn't even want to go to school, which in all other ways she loved. But what made up her mind to slim-down was wanting to find stylish clothes in which she'd look and feel comfortable; doing that had become increasingly difficult.

How Terri achieved her goal healthfully is what this chapter describes. You'll see how she tailored some of the many tips discussed earlier in order to manage her weight the right way. Essentially, Terri used the *pay for progress* strategy to move more, eat better, talk assertively, and avoid harm. At the end of the chapter, Terri talks about what the plan did *to* and *for* her.

Wanting their daughter to be happy and healthy, Terri's parents agreed to reward her for the next four months for carefully managing her weight. First, though, they had Terri visit their long-time family physician, Dr. Boyd. Going to the doctor had never been fun for Terri, but she did admire Dr. Boyd's skill, bedside manner, and sense of humor. Terri felt comfortable around Dr. Boyd, even though in the past had spilled many tears in the doctor's office. Dr. Boyd, however, could always cheer her up, making her laugh, and lately had inspired her to do well in school; Terri had decided to pursue a career in medicine.

Always welcoming, Dr. Boyd was especially happy that Terri wanted to no longer be overweight. Concerned that Terri had been gaining weight too fast the past year and would if nothing was done become obese, Dr. Boyd asked,

"Terri, why did you put on 20 pounds this past year?"

Shrugging her shoulders, Terri answered, "I don't know. I guess going from grade 8 to grade 9 was kind of scary. Anyway, I just got into the habit of eating lots of potato chips and candy and stuff like that after school. And I stopped skating and swimming, too."

"Terri becoming very heavy, obese, isn't the end of the world, but it does make slimming down much harder. So cut down on the snacking and start being active like before. Put the brakes on gaining weight. Just try not to gain for a while, and everything will be fine. But don't under any circumstances drastically diet, take diet pills, skip meals, or go on a fast. Don't try to lose weight. Let nature take its course, and you'll grow as you should without putting on pounds. Do that, and soon enough you'll no longer be overweight." (Terri liked the idea of losing overweight without actually having to lose weight.) "Call me if you have any questions. I want to see you in two months. By the way, here are two brochures, one on eating sensibly and the other on getting more active; they'll help you."

With that, Dr. Boyd gave Terri a big hug goodbye. Dr. Boyd also talked with Mrs. Melendez about what needed to happen and suggested ways to make it happen.

Two weeks later, after conferring with her parents and after some soul-searching and self-observation (see Tip # 1), Terri made her weight management plan. Her mom helped finalize it and write out its parts.

110

Terri's Weight Management Plan

PART ONE: The Goals

Terri decided upon these 8 goals

1) TO VISIT CHOOSEMYPLATE OFTEN

2) TO TAKE LESS FOOD (FEWER OR SMALLER HELPINGS) AT DINNER

3) TO STOP SUPERSIZING AT FAST FOOD RESTAURANTS

4) TO SNACK BETTER AT HOME (Terri snacked on many candy kisses and potato chips while in front of the TV and computer screen.)

5) TO PLAY MORE SPORTS (Terri rarely played team sports, preferring instead to watch TV or be on the computer).

6) TO WALK, SWIM, AND SKATE MORE

7) TO PRACTICE TALKING ASSERTIVELY (Lujane and Maggie teased Terri about her being heavy).

8) TO AVOID STRINGENT DIETING AND OTHER HARMFUL PRACTICES

PART TWO: THE RULES OF THE PLAN

When designing the plan, Terri and her parents agreed on:

1) HOW Terri WAS TO REACH EACH OF HER GOALS (Terri wrote down how she intended to reach each goal and the tip or tips showing her how.)

2) HOW MANY POINTS Terri WAS TO EARN FOR REACHING A SPECIFIC GOAL

3) HOW MUCH EACH REWARD POINT WAS TO BE WORTH (Each reward point was worth 20 cents.)

4) HOW Terri WAS TO USE THE CASH SHE RECEIVED FOR THE POINTS SHE EARNED (Terri decided to buy new clothes and some other items.)

5) HOW OFTEN Terri WAS TO CASH IN POINTS FOR MONEY

(Terri could trade her points for money whenever she wanted as long as she had the points first. That is, there would be no cash advances.)

6. HOW AND WHEN Terri's PROGRESS WAS TO BE CHECKED (Dr. Boyd or Terri would check Terri's BMI every two months. Online checkups could be done by visiting the BMI calculator webpage located at:

http://apps.nccd.cdc.gov/dnpabmi/Calculator.aspx)

PART THREE: REACHING GOALS AND EARNING POINTS

1. MY FIRST GOAL: Visit Choosemyplate in Order to Eat More Nutritiously

- HOW I INTEND TO REACH MY GOAL (tips #2, 3): I'll visit choosemyplate at least once every three weeks for about an hour to get information about nutritious foods and proper amounts for 14-year-olds.

- POINTS I'LL EARN FOR REACHING MY FIRST GOAL: 5 points for a one-hour visit to choosemyplate once every three weeks

2. MY SECOND GOAL : Take less at dinner

- HOW I INTEND TO REACH MY GOAL (tips #1, 8, 27, 33):. I'll take one less helping of dinner each night (tip #27). To do that, I'll count how many helpings I usually take of our usual dinners (tip #1) for one

112

week. Then, for the next several weeks, I'll take one less helping of those kinds of dinner.

- I'll slow my eating so that the helpings last longer (tip #33).

- If I want more, I'll substitute a plate of fruit for a second helping of the main dish. (tip #8)

- POINTS I'LL EARN FOR REACHING MY SECOND GOAL :5 points a week

3. MY THIRD GOAL: Stop Supersizing at fast food restaurants

- HOW I INTEND TO REACH MY GOAL (tips #26, 33)

- I'll ask for regular size hamburgers and fries and drinks at Fast Food restaurants. (tip #26)

- I'll plan what and how much I'll have there before I go

- I'll eat slower so that smaller sizes last longer and fill me up more (tip #33).

- POINTS I'LL EARN FOR REACHING MY THIRD GOAL: 10 points each time I don't supersize

4. MY FOURTH GOAL: Snack better at home

- HOW I INTEND TO REACH MY GOAL (tips #14,15,18, 21):

- I'll snack no more than once a week on potato chips. To do that, I'll get a container for snack-foods. I'll put one-half bag of potato chips in it, and put my name on the container (tip #18. Also, I'll substitute vegetables or fruit for all potato chip snacks but one (tip # 15).

- I'll stop snacking on candy kisses during the week. To help myself do that, I'll remove the candy dishes from the den where I usually snack (tip #21). Also, I'll make sure there are cut up vegetables in the refrigerator to substitute for the candy kisses (tips #14,15).

- POINTS I'LL EARN FOR REACHING MY FOURTH GOAL : 10 points per week

    a. 5 points when I don't snack on potato chips more than once per week

    b. 5 points when I don't snack on candy kisses during the week

5. MY FIFTH GOAL: Play more sports like basketball, badminton, volleyball, and soccer at school

- HOW I INTEND TO REACH MY GOAL(tip #36):

- I'll make sure I have runners, clean exercise clothes, a badminton racket, and two or three shuttlecocks at home. In this way I can bring what I need to school (tip #36).

- I'll arrange with Jen, Sal, Julie, Jeri, and Marci to play basketball, badminton, volleyball, or soccer. I'll also arrange to play on Monday, Wednesday, Thursday, and Friday (tip #36).

- POINTS I'LL EARN FOR REACHING MY FIFTH GOAL: 10 points for each hour I play

6. MY SIXTH GOAL: Walk or swim or skate more often

- HOW I INTEND TO REACH MY GOAL (tips #38,39):

- Swim on weekends an hour or so

- I'll walk Casey (Yorkshire terrier) at least once every day for about 20 minutes. Also, I'll do one of the following daily:

- I'll walk or skate to Jen's house, which is about 20 minutes away.

- I'll walk or skate about 20 minutes to shops on the corner for Mom.

- I'll skate for 30 minutes.

- POINTS I'LL EARN FOR REACHING MY SIXTH GOAL:

- 10 points for swimming about an hour or so

- 5 points for walking Casey about 20 minutes

- 5 points for walking or skating about 20 minutes without Casey to Jen's house or to stores on corner or for skating 30 minutes

7. MY SEVENTH GOAL: Talk assertively to Lujane and Maggie to stop their weight jokes and teasing

- HOW I INTEND TO REACH MY GOAL (tip #41):

- **First**, Diaphragm breathing. I'm already convinced I want to stand up for my rights. I'll practice diaphragm breathing

   1. I'll breathe-in so that my stomach moves out and then

   2. I'll breathe-out so that my stomach goes in

- **Second**, Calm myself before talking back. While breathing from the diaphragm, I'll practice calming myself. I'll breathe-in through my nose and hold my breath while I count to three. Then I'll breathe out with my lips pressed lightly together and say the word, relax, to myself. I'll practice breathing like this until I feel calm.

- **Third**, Practice alone how to talk assertively. I'll write out what I want to say to Lujane and Maggie. But I won't memorize it. I'll just be familiar with it. I'll use lots of "I feel" statements instead of "you did" ones. I'll practice alone in front of the mirror, making sure not to look away. I'll speak calmly, clearly, and friendly. I'll practice for a couple weeks or longer if I need to.

- **Fourth**, Practice with a friend how to talk assertively. I'll ask Marci to help me practice. First, Marci will pretend she's Lujane or Maggie while I'll play me. Then, I'll play Lujane or Maggie while Marci plays me. If Marci can't be my practice-partner, I'll ask Julie, Jen, Sal, or Jeri.

- **Fifth**, Talk assertively to Lujane and Maggie. When I'm comfortable, I'll talk assertively to Lujane. Then, later, I'll talk assertively to Maggie.

- POINTS I'LL EARN FOR REACHING MY SEVENTH GOAL:

    20 points for practicing alone or with a friend

    25 points for talking assertively to Lujane

    25 points for talking assertively to Maggie

8. MY EIGHTH GOAL: Avoid Harm

- HOW I INTEND TO REACH MY GOAL (tips #43-52):

- I'll avoid the temptation to stringently diet, fast, skip meals, and so on by thinking about what I've learned from Dr. Boyd and Mrs. Schott, my gym teacher.

- POINTS I'LL EARN FOR REACHING MY EIGHTH GOAL: 5 points per week for behaving sensibly

PART FOUR: THE PRIZES Terri COULD BUY

In her diary, Terri kept track of the points she earned. She traded them for cash every couple of weeks. In the first column that follows are the items she could buy with the cash. In the second column are the costs of these items in points and real money.

ITEMS	COST: Points/Money
cell phone	500 = $100
White blouse	200 = $40
netbook computer	2000 = $400
Lined Jeans	190 = $38
Regular Jeans	200 = $40
New runners	500 = $100
New boots	600 = $120
1 CD	90 = $18
1 DVD	100 = $20
Pink Sleep-shirt	80= $16
Gray Cardigan	330 = $66
Wool Sweater	400 = $80
Warm-up Suit	500 = $100

PART FIVE: SPONSORS' PLEDGE TO PAY TERRI FOR HER PROGRESS:

Parents pledge to give Terri 20 cents ($.20) for each point she earns. She can exchange points for money whenever she chooses provided she has the points.

PART SIX: SIGNATURES

I agree to do my best to manage my weight.

Signature: Terri Melendez

We, Terri's parents, agree to finance this pay for progress

Signature: A. Melendez   Signature:
R. Melendez

~~

Terri's four-month weight management plan worked wonderfully for her. She had this to say about it:

"When I decided to do something about my weight, I was in the lunchroom at the table with Lujane and her friends. Sometimes Lujane really makes me mad. She thinks she's so cool. She thinks anyone who doesn't look like she believes they're supposed to look isn't cool. She and Maggie tease me about my weight—they think they're funny, but I don't. It hurts. That's a big reason why I made up my mind to do something about my weight, but it wasn't the only reason. I also wanted to be able to find popular styles to wear that I looked good in and that fit comfortably.

I didn't want to make a big production out of this weight thing. It's nobody's business but mine, and I'm not going to advertise that I'm too heavy by telling everyone I'm doing something about being heavy. That's kind of like saying there's a problem. And I know somebody, sometime, would joke about it. But I did want mom and dad to help, and they asked Dr. Boyd to get involved, too, so I did go a little public. Nobody at school except Marci knew at the start what I was doing, and she promised to keep quiet about it.

I wasn't sure the weight management plan Dr. Boyd, my parents, and I came up with would work. I didn't know if I could follow it, and I didn't want to fail. Then, Dr. Boyd told me that if it didn't work for me, it didn't mean I was a failure. It just meant I should keep trying to find a plan that would work.

That made me feel better, so I decided to give weight management a try. Once I got going, it wasn't that hard, actually kind of fun, especially when I got points and saw that I could do it. When something didn't work, I either changed it or looked for something better. When things did go right, I felt great. Getting reward points was nice, too.

Playing volleyball is more fun than I thought it would be. I even liked walking Casey.

I can boss my own eating/snacking now more than before, and that feels good. Really like that my clothes look and fit better, too. There's lots to pick from now.

It's great that I talked back to Lujane and Maggie. That part of the plan scared me the most. However, during a progress check, Dr. Boyd helped me figure out what to say to them. I practiced what we decided, first alone and then with Marci, but still was nervous right before I met with Lujane. It went okay though. I told her that her teasing and weight jokes bothered me and that it was unfair. She listened. I tried not to sound angry or sorry for myself but just said how I felt. Maybe we'll never be good friends again, but she's been nicer. I talked to Maggie, too, and said almost the same things to her but don't think she really cared that much. She hasn't been too bad lately though, so maybe she did listen a little.

My biggest problem in living up to the weight management plan was wanting it to work fast. Sometimes I was tempted to really cut calories, but knew from Dr. Boyd and Mrs. Schott, my gym teacher, what doing that could cause. So I tried to be more patient.

I'm glad I followed my weight management plan and will do so again. Hope it continues working."

~~

It did. Feeling happy and motivated because it did, Terri stayed in charge of her weight every day, making several other similar weight management deals with her parents over the year. By her 15th birthday, she had reached a healthy weight for her height. As Dr. Boyd had predicted, simply by putting the brakes on gaining while growing during the year — Terri grew 3 inches— the teen had lowered her body mass index from 26.4 to 23.9. She was no longer overweight.

~~

Weight management plans like these add a little competition and fun to the weight management job. Successfully following them gets you money, cell phones, new clothes, and other desirables. Much more important though, successfully following them boosts your chances of having good health and feelings of well-being that last.

Chapter 14
Cautions & Tips in a Nutshell

Remember the first time you sat on a two wheel bike? Probably you were nervous, maybe scared to death. Even if the outstretched arms of someone you trusted were there, you likely still had butterflies in your stomach.

Remember the first day at the school you're attending? Were you a bundle of nerves? Did you get lost in the halls, forget your locker combination, mispronounce your teacher's name, believe no one liked you? Or did you just worry such things would happen? No matter if real or imagined, all of that is probably behind you by now, just bad memories. What was new and upsetting on day 1 has become familiar and routine thanks to time, practice, and experience.

Keep that in mind if today you think that managing your weight will be like climbing a mountain tomorrow. It won't be. Instead, it will be like riding a bike or navigating somewhere new. Time, practice, and experience will prove it's not too hard, complicated, and interfering.

~~

So, try it. Deciding to manage your weight could be one of the most life- enhancing, life-preserving decisions you'll ever make. This book will help you do this vital job well. Here again are some cautions to remember and 52 tips to consider as you forge ahead.

BEFORE ATTEMPTING TO MANAGE YOUR WEIGHT

1. Talk with Your Parents about Your Intentions

2. Talk with the Family Doctor about Your Intentions Including Whether You Should or Should Not Lose Weight

121

3. Accept Responsibility for the Weight Management Job

4. Commit to Trying Hard to Do the Job Well

WHILE ATTEMPTING TO MANAGE YOUR WEIGHT

5. Seek Nutritious Foods & Nutritional Bargains & Don't Diet Unless a Doctor or Dietitian Says to

6. Seek Support from Others like Parents & Friends

7. Avoid the Snakes of Weight Mismanagement (Tips #43-52)

8. Be Patient and Gradual When Making Changes

FIFTY-TWO TIPS FOR CORRECTLY MANAGING WEIGHT

LOCATING EATING HOTSPOTS

#1 Shine a Light on Your Eating.

CHOOSING FOODS & MEALS

#2 Explore Choosemyplate.

#3 Interact with Choosemyplate.

#4 Eat Breakfast, Lunch, and Dinner Each Day.

#5 Go to Fast-Food Restaurants Less Often.

#6 Plan What You'll Order Before Going to a Fast Food Restaurant.

#7 Baked and Broiled Foods Are Better for You than Fried Foods.

#8 For Dessert Sometimes Substitute Fresh Fruit for Pie, Cake, Cookies, and Ice Cream.

#9 Drink Water More Often & Sugary Soft Drinks Less Often.

#10 Eat More Vegetables and Salad At Dinner.

SNACKING SMARTER

#11 Trick Some of Your Snack Attacks.

#12 Have the Right Number of Nutritious Snacks.

#13 Ask Your Parents to Keep Less Candy and Fewer Salty High-in-Fat Snack-foods, like Potato Chips, at Home.

#14 Ask Your Parents to Keep Many Fruits and Cut Vegetables on Hand for Snacks.

#15 Have More Fruit, Raw Vegetables or Cereal When Snacking Instead of Candy, Cookies, and Chips.

#16 Make Snacks More Chewy by Adding Vegetables or Fruit To Them So They Last Longer..

#17 Have a Special Place to Snack At Home.

#18 Have Your Own (with your name on it) Snack Box At Home.

#19 Remove Food from Your Bedroom; Too Easy To Snack There

#20 Remove Food from Your School Locker.

#21 Ask Your Parents to Remove Any Candy Dishes Placed Near the TV or Computer.

#22 Snack Less or Not At All While Watching Television or When at the Computer.

#23 Don't Snack (& Fill-up) On Bread While Waiting For Dinner At Restaurants.

#24 Don't Buy Snack Foods and Soft Drinks from Vending Machines.

#25 Ask Friends, Grandparents, Aunts, and Uncles Not to Offer You So Many Candies, Chips, Cookies, Cakes, and Foods Like Them To Snack On.

RETRAINING YOUR BRAIN TO EAT LESS

#26 Retrain Your Brain To Take Smaller Portions at Home & Restaurants.

#27 Retrain Your Brain To Take Fewer Helpings.

#28 Retrain Your Brain To Eat When Hungry, Stop When Full.

#29 Let Moderate Not Intense Hunger Guide You.

#30, Don't Purposely Starve During the Day in Order to Stuff at Night.

#31 Don't Eat Just Because Foods You See On TV Plead, "Try Me You'll Love Me."

#32 Don't Eat Just Because Others Are Eating.

#33 Eat Slower and Chew More Thoroughly To Feel Fuller.

ACTIVITY: ACTIVATING, PLANNING, DOING, STAYING

#34 Get At Least Sixty Minutes of Moving-more Activity Each Day, Every day.

#35 Find out Your Activity-likes.

#36 Make A Weekly Activity Plan.

#37 Pay for Progress.

#38 Make Being Active Fun.

#39 Be Active in Many Ways, But Don't Overdo It.

40 Make Rainy Day Activity Plans. Don't Let Bad Weather Keep You Idle.

THINKING UPBEAT THOUGHTS & TALKING BACK TO YOURSELF

#41 Talk back to Those Who Bring You Down: Others & Yourself.

STIMULUS CONTROL

#42 Practice Good Stimulus Control of Your Eating & Activity.

SNAKES

#43 Don't Seek the Miracle Cure. Abracadabra and....

#44 Don't Take Non-prescription Diet Pills.

#45 Don't Become A Slave to Weight Scales by Over checking Your Weight

#46 Don't Fast or Skip Meals.

#47 Don't Purposely Purge.

#48 Don't Put Too Much on the Line.

#49 Don't Give Up On Trying to Help Yourself.

#50 Don't Think What You Weigh Is Who You Are.

#51 Don't Count Calories Obsessively.

#52 Don't Make "Never Again Promises" about So-called Forbidden Foods.

~~

Feel free to write to me if you have any questions about anything in this book. I will do my best to answer in a timely fashion. My e-mail address is: mlebow@cc.umanitoba.ca.

Good luck.

Chapter 15
For Parents

This book tells adolescents what overweight and obesity mean, do not mean, and mindful of how fragile a heavy teenager's self-esteem can be, should never mean. As well, *the book* offers its young readers healthy weight management alternatives to unhealthy weight- control practices, practices that unfortunately many young people often resort to. Over the years, my teenage clients have asked me most of the questions this book poses. I hope your sons and daughters and you, too, feel I've answered them well.

There's one question more to address: how can parents help their overweight/obese adolescent children. The task of assisting them can be frustrating and daunting, but certainly is doable. The pages to follow describe some helping essentials.

REMAIN MINDFUL OF FEELINGS AND BE SUPPORTIVE

Above all, you want your children to feel worthwhile, accepted, supported, understood, and valued. Easy to say. But if their environment regularly and callously tramples their self-esteem, hard to ensure. Too often teenagers with weight problems have to contend with:

- bullies at home and at school who ridicule the heavy

- peers who demand *be thin to be in*

- friends and family members who say, "you'd look better if thinner"

- media that revere thin bodies and lampoon heavy ones

- teachers who publicly warn of the perils of being overweight/obese

Nevertheless not all heavy teenagers having to face such unfriendly environments will seek or accept their parents' weight management advice. If your offer of help is rejected, what then can you do? If you decide to just hope that time will erase the problem — wait-and-see — know that your decision is risky. That's because if left untreated, many overweight/obese teenagers become overweight/obese adults, spend their adolescent years miserable, or in desperation try dangerous weight-loss stratagems. There is, however, one thing you can do that could benefit your heavy teenager and everyone else in the family as well: make a few easy-to-tolerate healthier-living home improvements. For example:

1. *Encourage the family to exercise together.* Planned weekend bike rides and trips to the local indoor or outdoor pool or, depending on the climate where you live, snowshoeing, cross-country skiing, skateboarding, tennis, volleyball, and badminton are just some of the ways to get everyone in the family moving more. Whatever you choose, make certain the family has the equipment and apparel needed for the family exercise days.

2. *Stockpile fewer high calorie, high-fat snacks.*

3. *Store hard-to-resist leftovers in hard-to-see-through.containers.*

4. *Stockpile nutritional bargains.* Foods like fruits and vegetables are nutritional bargains, providing more nutrition calorie for calorie than most other foods do.

5. *Create well-balanced meals that include the recommended food groups.* The best source of information for doing that is the food guide at www.choosemyplate.gov. Replete with time-saving tips and innovative suggestions, this website is a treasure chest.

A caution. When you try to improve the family's dietary habits, go slowly or risk much grumbling and resistance; granted, sometimes medical reasons demand that changes be speedy, but that's unusual. In addition to going slowly, request everyone's input. Solicited changes made gradually work better and last longer than imposed ones made suddenly.

6. *Ask heavy teenagers to help plan family menus.*

7. *Ask grandparents and other relatives who overfeed to stop it.*

8. *Ask siblings who tease their heavy brothers or sisters about being heavy to stop it.* Reward them for teasing less with more say over what goes into their personal snack-food containers.

9. *Don't make heavy teenagers into dietary outcasts.* Prepare the same foods for everyone unless a doctor or dietitian prescribes a special diet for your overweight/obese adolescent.

10. *Pay for progress when asked to.* The pay for progress method boosts morale and motivation. It's sometimes the only way heavy teenagers will start and stay on the road to eating smarter and moving more (see tip #37).

11. *Help expose eating hotspots when asked* to. Eating hotspots are specific practices and routines interfering with smarter eating (see tip #1). Uncover them to overcome them.

12. *Remove the weight management contradictions present in your home.* Such disagreements exist when what you do or say concerning food conflicts with what you do or say concerning weight. The following recollection of a previously overweight teenager who's now a thin adult illustrates the **food is splendor but heaviness is ugly** contradiction.

"I remember that dinners during the work-week were superior: meat (brisket), never less than two of cooked vegetables (cooked with lots of butter and love), some raw carrots and celery (but who wanted them?), potatoes fried crisply, sometimes rice, sometimes both. Pie, for afterwards, never naked on the plate was adorned with ice cream (sometimes ice milk because it sounded low-cal). The food parade never ended. We usually sat down at six o'clock and began eating when we saw our filled plates. I always ate all the visible reasons on mine to continue eating, refilling or stopping only when the food vanished. Rarely was I only satisfied, never was I left hungry. To be full was to be bloated. Indeed, during my childhood and my adolescence food was love, and eating was ecstasy."

Now, the contradiction:

"I clearly recall that my mother and father touted anti-fat propaganda as much as anyone could. Also critical of extra poundage, my grandparents joined with them in repeatedly warning that heaviness, ugliness, and weakness shared the same seat at the dinner table."

The food is splendor but heaviness is ugly inconsistency

This compromises the efforts of teenagers trying to battle weight problems. Ease their burden, and remove this confusing contradiction if you find it in your home.

The next contradiction, **"clean your plate if you want dessert, but stop eating so many sweets"** also roadblocks smarter eating. Its rationale that food is too precious to waste is sensible. But its remedy that wasting can be stopped by rewarding continued eating with rich desserts is illogical, particularly when directed at heavy young people who have been or soon will be admonished for overeating sweets.

13. *Serve less, waste less.* To combat food-wasting, it's better to offer heavy teenagers less food than to bargain with them to eat more.

14. *Promote the natural reasons to eat.* Eat when hungry, stop when full. Hunger and satiety, the internal regulators of our

130

eating that we are born with, work for us in the long run better than the external cues to eat like rich food displays (tip #28).

15. *Make weight management a family affair.* This could involve two or more family members practicing the tips this book offers. Or relatedly it could involve you and your heavy teenager together reading this book or one like it.

These 15 suggestions, some small and some large, have only sampled the improvements parents can sponsor. Before implementing any be certain your teenagers know about and agree with them. By giving your sons and daughters a voice in deciding what will happen, you increase the likelihood they'll view the eventual changes as supportive instead of as controlling.

TALK TO THE DOCTOR

For teenagers,medical input is a "must-have" part of all weight management programs before beginning them and throughout. The doctor can do many things for heavy teenagers including:

- *Checking their health status.* Likely this will include searching for disease risk factors such as high blood pressure, high triglycerides, and insulin resistance and for obesity-related diseases like type II diabetes.

- *Calculating their body mass index (BMI).* Teenagers as well can track their BMI changes online at http://apps.nccd.cdc.gov/dnpabmi/ Calculator.aspx

- *Interpreting their body mass index.* This involves comparing the heavy teenager's BMI to the BMI representative of others the teenager's age and sex— his or her reference group. A teenager is overweight when 85% to under 95% of others in the reference group have a lower BMI and obese when 95% or more of them do.

- *Determining their daily calorie needs* (see also tip #3)

- *Determining their immediate and future weight goals.* The goals are either growing without gaining, growing and gaining little, or losing small amounts of weight gradually.

- *Determining their nutritional* needs. The doctor might recommend consulting a dietitian to do that.

- *Prescribing necessary and proscribing unnecessary behavioral changes.* The doctor might recommend consulting a behavioral specialist to help do this.

CREATE THE CLIMATE TO COMMUNICATE

Talk to your teenagers about healthy weight management. Are they clear about the wrong ways and the right ways to go about it, and are they clear about what to expect?

The chances you'll get frank answers to such questions and be seen as an ally increase if the climate of communication is good. Unfortunately, there is no blueprint to ensure it will be good, but there are a few do's and don'ts to be mindful of when trying to make it better. They are:

Avoid communication turnoffs

Blaming and shaming, interrogating and commanding, ordering and threatening, lecturing and preaching interfere with satisfying exchanges. Anyone who employs any of these turnoffs is easier to avoid than talk with.

Speak with "I's"

Want Jo to know your viewpoint without getting defensive if it questions hers, reveal what you have to say with "I" statements.

132

"Jo, I realize that sometimes it's easier just to eat nothing at all than to eat less, but I do worry when you fast to control your weight. I know it's unhealthy, and I've read it just makes a person hungrier. I'd feel better if we'd find another way."

The alternative is to "you" her.

"Jo, you shouldn't fast. If you do, you're jeopardizing yourself. Fasting just makes you hungrier and heavier. Think about it Jo, you're doing something dangerous and silly."

"I" statements further communication. "You" ones stop it, especially when they accuse, blame, or shame.

Show you're tuned-in

Valuable in revealing you're listening and understanding are rephrasing what's been said, asking for clarification when needed, keeping eye contact, and validating by agreeing with what's been said when you do agree.

Listen empathically

Here's what I **don't** mean:

Mom: "Hi Honey, bad day?" (Good opening)

Sean: "I really hate it there. Midland High sucks. Just fat jokes all day long. Not worth it. Home-schooling or going back to my old school for one more year would be better than this. Maybe a job, I'm almost 18. I should leave."

Mom: "Don't be ridiculous. It's a hard world for anyone without an education. You leave, you'll find out. You're almost ready for college, so why stop now. We've spent a lot to live here, just so you could go to Midland. That's the best place if you want to go to college. Just forget about the weight teasing."

Sean: "College's not everything."

Mom: "You should just go to Midland each day. Ignore the teasing, and remember the sacrifices our family's made so you can get a good education. You know what that means to us and Grandpa. Think you're the only one with a high school nightmare? Check with Grandpa about what I had to go through, and I didn't drop out and let him down."

Sean: "I'm not you Mom. What's for dinner?"

Conversation over. Mom replies to Sean with her perspective before understanding his. She thinks: *I know what I'm saying makes sense. I'll never understand why he just won't listen to me.* But Mom, as Dr. Stephen Covey in *7 habits of highly effective people* would observe, has the communication problem somewhat backwards. Sean won't listen to her because she won't listen to him. For Sean to understand Mom, even though he may disagree with her, she needs to show that she understands him. She has to listen to him—his pain, his confusion, his desires. In Covey's words, *Seek first to understand then to be understood* (p. 237).

Let's replay Sean's and Mom's conversation, but with Mom now listening to Sean's feelings and viewpoint.

Mom: "Hi Honey, bad day?"

Sean: "I really hate it there. Midland High really sucks. Just fat jokes all day long. Not worth it. Home schooling or going back to my old school for one more year would be better than this. Maybe a job, I'm almost 18. I should leave."

Mom: "Guess you're feeling awful there."

Sean: "Yeah, it's really getting to me."

Mom: "Sounds like you've had it and need a change."

134

This instead of telling Sean to ignore difficulties, to focus on college, and to please parents and Grandpa. And this instead of attempting to guilt and shame Sean.

> **Sean**: "I'm scared of changing. I know I have only a few more months, and I know graduating from Midland will help me get into college. You and Dad have laid out a bundle to live here, so I can go to Midland, but they just won't leave me alone."

> **Mom**: "Sometimes it must be hard for you even to breathe there, like you're being choked and want to escape, right?"

> **Sean**: "Right. But I want to go to a good college and not disappoint you and Dad. What should I do?"

Conversation far from over. Mom's empathic responding has created a warm safe environment for Sean to open up in and explain himself. Likely, he will see her as trying to understand his plight. If instead Sean believes she doesn't appreciate his problems, he won't seek her counsel. He won't talk more, he won't share more, he won't risk more, he won't listen more. Things he must do if Mom is to know what he wants and what advice she should give him, advice he may eventually reject, but at least now be more likely to hear.

Keep in mind that empathic listening means nothing if your teenagers see you as phony, artificial, or duplicitous. Your sincerity, genuineness, and caring are critical and their trust in you essential before they'll share. How do you communicate these positive qualities to your sons and daughters? Dr. Covey would say by your character: by truly being sincere, genuine, trustworthy, and caring in all that you do.

~~

To help your heavy teenagers accept your help, speak well and listen well.

136

References

Covey, S. R. *The 7 habits of highly effective people* (1989). New York: Simon &Schuster.

Centers for Disease Control and Prevention: Activity for Everyone: Introduction. This site provides information on measuring the intensity of physical activity, what fitness is all about, tips on the beginning an activity regimen, and a wealth of other valuable information for bringing activity into your life.

Link: http://www.cdc.gov/nccdphp/dnpa/physical/index.htm

Centers for Disease Control and Prevention: body mass index. This site offers a multitude of links to all sorts of body mass index information including computation and interpretation.

Link: http://www.cdc.gov/nccdphp/dnpa/bmi/

Centers for Disease Control and Prevention: Body and mind website: this site provides a wealth of tips on finding activity likes.

Link: www.bam.gov/index.html

Centers for Disease Control and Prevention: Overweight and Obesity. This comprehensive link from the(CDC) answers many questions about overweight and obesity. Numerous links are embedded in it, including one that addresses issues pertinent to childhood and adolescent overweight and obesity.

Link: http://www.cdc.gov/nccdphp/dnpa/obesity/

Choosemyplate (2012). This is one of the best dietary systems for the whole family. Children, teenagers, and adults learn what and how much of what to eat. The choosemyplate system was established in 2012. It has proven to be valuable in fulfilling its mandate of improving what Americans eat. The choosemyplate site provides numerous links to a wealth of information on nutrition and energy needs.

Link: http://www.choosemyplate.gov

Davis, J. (1980). *Garfield at large: his first book*. New York: Ballantine Books.

Grand, L.C. (2000). *The Marriage & Family Presentation Guide.* New York: John Wiley & Sons, Inc.

Grosko, T.(2008). *Obesity Stigma Reduction.* Unpublished doctoral dissertation.

Leahy, R. & Holland, S. (2000). *Treatment Plans and Interventions for depression and anxiety disorders.* New York: Guilford

LeBow, M. D. (1995). *Overweight teenagers: Don't bear the burden alone.* New York: Plenum (Insight Books).

Thomas, G. (1986). *Leader effectiveness Training* New York: Bantam Doubleday Dell.

Thouas, L. (2008). *The use of empathy interventions in reducing obesity stigmatization.* Unpublished master's thesis.

Index

A

Activating(see also moving more)

Q

Questions

Tips,52 (listed)   **122-125**

Tips Discussed

Also by Michael LeBow from Science & Humanities Press

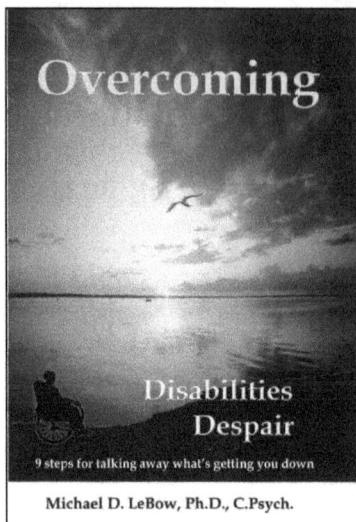

Overcoming Disabilities Despair

Life gives everybody things they can't control. Sometimes, even the most capable and productive people hit against a personal limitation and get discouraged over things they can't do.

So what do you do when life hands you a major setback? Do you quit, sink into despair and wait for something good to happen to get you past the depression? This book offers practical help from a well-known expert who understands disabilities from his own personal experiences.

Educators & Seniors Discount Policy

To encourage use of our books for education, educators can purchase three or more books (mixed titles) on our standard discount schedule for resellers. See

sciencehumanitiespress.com/educator/educator.html

for more detail.

Science & Humanities Press

PO Box 7151

Chesterfield MO 63006-7151

www.ingramcontent.com/pod-product-compliance
Lightning Source LLC
Chambersburg PA
CBHW072252270326
41930CB00010B/2356